Wisdom For Health

6 WEEK LOW CARB DIET
With
Intermittent Fasting

Achieve your ideal weight, regain energy, live longer, look fantastic and learn to create yummy and healthy foods.

Other books by: Philip Bridgeman

- Daniels Diet
- Daniel's Diet Recipe Guide
- Daniel's Diet Lifestyle
- Are You Tired, Lethargic and Can't Lose Weight (EBook)
- Quick and Easy Meals (EBook)
- 5 Common Foods that Causes Bloated Stomach and Embarrassing Flatulence (EBook)

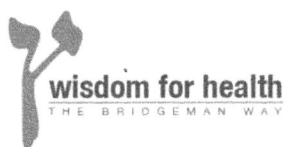

Copyright Notices
Copyright © 2023 Philip Bridgeman
Email: **philip@optusnet.com.au**
Website: **www.wisdomforhealth.com**

All rights reserved. No part of this publication may be reproduced, stored in a retrieval system or transmitted in any form or by any means electronic, mechanical, photocopying, recording or otherwise without the prior written permission of the publisher.

Disclaimer:

This book is not intended to take the place of or give medical advice or treatment. Readers are advised to consult their own doctor regarding the treatment of their medical problems. People with serious health issues should be under professional supervision before attempting this diet. All the names of people used as case histories have been changed to protect their privacy. The success stories from people who have completed this diet are individual cases and do not guarantee that you will get the same results. This book is based on the personal clinical experience of the author. Neither the publisher, the author, nor anyone involved in this book's creation takes any responsibility for possible consequences caused by any treatment, action or application of any herb, diet or preparation used by any person.

Publisher – PK Self Publishers
Website: www.pkselfpublishers.com
Email: admin@pkselfpublishers.com

DO YOU WANT TO...

- Lose weight & remain healthy?
- Keep the weight off?
- Stop feeling hungry?
- Stop craving sugar?
- Overcome emotional eating?
- Regain energy & make the most out of your life.

This diet (eating) plan has helped many people lose weight and regain their health. It's been tried and tested with incredible results for over 20 years in clinical and group use.

I can confidently and unequivocally state that this diet plan works – How? Because of the thousands of success stories I have witnessed.

Nutritionist, Naturopath, Herbalist, Life Coach & Award Winning Author Philip Bridgeman, ND. BSc.

Authors Introduction

With so many products and weight loss systems in the marketplace, how do you decide what is right for you? Nearly every person over 15 years old has tried a **diet** of some description; people often say to me, "You name the diet, and I've tried it", and "Please help me; I just can't lose weight no matter what I try?"

There is always an answer, and I encourage you not to give up even if you have tried nearly every diet known to humankind. All you need is a plan that you can trust and that suits you, and I aim to supply you with that plan based on 30 years of successful clinical experience.

Why is it so hard? Why all the different opinions?

The Diet Plan I have successfully used for many years that I now present to you is the answer and vital to weight loss and overcoming health issues. As a health practitioner, my calling in life is to teach and help people lose weight and live a healthy, long life. Over many years of practice, I have used all sorts of diets and fasting techniques, so I have put together a gold star system that allows you to benefit from my clinical knowledge.

This 6-week Diet is not a long-term plan; it is designed to be used in blocks of 6 weeks and in a rotational method with my joint diet plan, Daniels Diet.

The two-step Weight Loss Plan.

My unique weight loss plan, which I refined in my clinical practice over many years, works like this:

Phase one, which you follow for ten days, is called the **Daniels Diet**. This Diet I based on the biblical book of Daniel, chapter one. The Daniels Diet cuts out all processed foods and all grains; you eat only fruits & veggies. It centres around eating any food grown in our 'Gods Garden', i.e., only naturally grown foods, meaning it is a vegetarian and vegan diet. It is gluten-free and Dairy free.

Phase Two is the 6-Week Low-Carb Diet.

These two diets are very different; however, they have profound results if used separately. Together they give you two different methods with various food choices that suit everyone. The two plans synchronise and work exceptionally well to help you lose weight and regain energy.

Summary of the two weight loss plans: start with either method and rotate at the appropriate times. For example, you complete the 6-week low-carb Diet and immediately change to the 10-day Daniels Diet or vice versa. You can alternate them several times if need be to reach your weight loss goals.

When you have reached your goals, you can blend the two and have a healthy lifestyle eating plan in the longer term and, of course, with the occasional day out for celebrations.

Note: You can repeat both diets on and off for the rest of your life.

- So I encourage you - Do not let past diet negative experiences stop you from seeking the answers and finding the eating plan that suits you in the short and long term!
- Decide to commit to this program and expect good results. Think, talk, expect and picture (imagine) a successful and enjoyable journey ahead of you.
- If you speak negatively about yourself, your body shape and eating habits, change to positive faith-filled words and see what God will do.

Table of Contents

DO YOU WANT TO 4

AUTHORS INTRODUCTION 5

CHAPTER ONE 9

An Easy-to-Follow Weight Loss Program 9
    Welcome 10
    To the 6-week Low Carb and High Protein Diet. 10

CHAPTER TWO 13

The Secret to This Diet Plan! 13
    Exercise is a key! 14

CHAPTER THREE 17

Set Your Personal Goals 17
    The Goals of This 6-Week Healthy Eating Planner 19
    What Are the Benefits for Me? 19
    Motivation & Help for Emotional Eating. 20

CHAPTER FOUR 23

The Shopping List 23
    Meats 24
    Vegetable Oils 25
    Beverages 25
    Not Allowed Food 27

CHAPTER FIVE 30

Intermittent Fasting (IF) 30
    My IF program. 32
    BREAKFAST RECIPES 34
    Snacks RECIPES 47

CHAPTER SIX 55

LUNCHES / DINNER 55
Salad Bar 59
Fish and *Seafood* 63
Tuna Pie 72
Chicken 74
Turkey 87
Beef 89

CHAPTER SEVEN 95

This Diet Plan Makes Socialising Easy and Enjoyable. 95

SUMMARY: 97

ABOUT THE AUTHOR 98

Chapter One

An Easy-to-Follow Weight Loss Program

Weight loss is a vitally important subject and not just a cosmetic issue. It is vital for self-image, self-esteem, and to look your best. However, it goes way beyond that – why? **Because the contribution of obesity to ill health is now greater than that of tobacco smoking.**

Obesity is a significant driver in many health problems people face. Losing just 3 kilos could dramatically lower your chance of developing certain diseases.

This 6-week diet plan is designed to assist you in losing up to 2 kg of fat per week whilst preserving your muscle mass. Most calorie-restricted diets produce disappointing results due to the excessive loss of muscle mass. The loss of muscle may reduce your metabolic rate (ability to burn calories) and increases the possibility of putting the fat back on (yo-yo dieting).

This diet plan will help you avoid the damaging effects of yo-yo dieting. Gain long-term results and receive knowledge and understanding on creating the body you want to see and the 'Health' you want to feel.

Welcome

To the 6-week Low Carb and High Protein Diet.

The low-fat – high carbohydrate diets used in the past failed to prevent obesity. In fact, over the last 30 years, total fat intake has decreased, yet obesity is increasing to epidemic proportions.

Low carbohydrate diets have been more effective and provide substantial additional benefits beyond fat reduction and the treatment of overweight and obesity.

The Added Benefits of this Diet Plan:

1. Obesity is a risk factor for many chronic diseases, such as cardiovascular diseases, type-2 diabetes, cancer and arthritis. Losing weight has been demonstrated to reduce the risk of developing these chronic diseases.

2. I have noticed these Diets can help with anxiety and melancholic depression. This eating system may be used to reduce obesity and improve your moods.

3. The Diet plan may also help balance excess oestrogen levels.

Obesity is typically associated with elevated oestrogen levels. The more fat you have, the more your body can create oestrogen, (oestrogen has been given to animals to fatten them up quickly?) It has been called 'the fat hormone'.

This imbalance occurs due to elevated insulin levels from having a high sugar and highly refined carbohydrate diet in the past, associated with insulin resistance and obesity, which inhibit the conversion of androgens to oestrogen in the ovaries. Using this type of diet system may reduce this conversion.

This low carbohydrate plan is one of the most successful fat-reducing programs I have used in 30 years of clinical practice.

- The program offers you many tasty and easy-to-follow recipes.

- Because it has lots of protein – it satisfies your hunger, and many people will agree to follow it as you should not feel hungry. You can eat meat.

It will help anyone with insulin resistance (sugar issues) –which is one of the key factors for anyone who finds it hard to lose weight.

Chapter Two

The Secret to This Diet Plan!

How to Dissolve Your Body Fat?

Nature (God) has provided us with three primary sources of energy. Our body can burn stored fat, glucose (carbohydrate), or protein for energy. If you eat less carbohydrate than you require for energy output, your stored fat is burned to satisfy your body's energy requirements.

This means you should lose weight because there are only three main fuel systems your body draws on, and the idea is to restrict the one, which is carbohydrates, and your body then has to burn the second one (fat) for energy. Keep in mind that most people overeat refined carbohydrates in their daily diet, leading to obesity over years of eating like this. This is why many people' yo-yo' Diet; the minute they finish any diet plan, they return to old habits and eat what they are habitually used to (too many sugars and carbohydrates) and put all the weight back on.

The modern diet is full of high glycaemic load foods, i.e. sugar (or refined carbs). Food such as starchy, highly processed bread, packet cereal, white flour products, cakes, cookies (biscuits), ice cream, pastry, pasta, white rice, fast foods, don't forget alcohol and sugary products such as soft drinks, cordials and reconstituted fruit juices which are all quickly converted by your body into glucose.

High amounts of glucose will cause the release of high doses of insulin, encouraging your body to store these carbohydrate foods as fat and stop fat from being used as energy (therefore increasing weight gain). It becomes challenging to lose fat if you have raised insulin levels.

When your body's blood sugar and insulin levels are low enough, you will switch to a higher level of fat burning. **The secret to this Diet is to diminish your sugar/ carb intake and trigger off burning fat, and you lose weight. Remember t**o burn fat, you need to restrict highly refined Carbohydrates (i.e. glycaemic load) foods to an amount where your body will produce less insulin, thereby increasing the fat-burning rate. Eating less food is not the answer; you need to specifically reduce the high glycaemic index and carbohydrate-rich foods in order to 'switch on' fat burning. Also, by the end of the 6 weeks, your taste buds should have lost the cravings for sugar (refined carbs).

I suggest you request a fasting insulin resistance blood test next time you visit your local doctor. This test is specific for insulin resistance and different to the blood glucose test. If you find it hard to lose weight, this may be the reason. There are lovely herbs that go along with the Diets to help you if your test shows you are insulin resistant.

Exercise is a key!
There are no shortcuts. No one can do it for you, and it must be done, so decide to get in the habit regularly and enjoy. If you exercise before a meal, this will allow your body to burn the stored fat as well and help you lose weight. Exercise has many health benefits, including aiding digestion and bowel movements (regular bowel movements are vital for health and weight loss – at least once daily).

After exercising, it's wise to eat something nutritious within half an hour of completion as you need to replace lost energy and prevent the overwhelming cravings for sugar or carbs' that often drive us to head for chocolate or a sweet fix. Eat protein or have a whey protein shake.

Increasing weight-bearing exercise as well as aerobics is a very beneficial plan. This gives you more muscle mass and will increase your metabolism.

A higher metabolic rate helps lessen the chance of weight gain and obesity throughout life. Also, fun and active outings decrease boredom and make time available for extra snacking or grazing at home. It will also help boost self-esteem, and if you are an emotional eater, this is a big help. Your goals need to be; realistic, enjoyable, specific, and positive.

I found a basic heart rate monitor helpful because it showed me that I was not exercising adequately. It gave me new goals to reach. In fact, my heart rate was way too low to burn up enough energy to lose weight effectively.

You see, it's best to keep your heart rate up to a certain level (if needed, get professional help to know where your rate should be) and keep it there for 30 – 45 minutes at a time; then, you will see better results. Also, I learnt that it's more effective to vary the intensity of aerobic exercise from moderate to high during the workout. Regular exercise is the best way to maintain healthy body weight and increase your energy levels.

Exercise should raise your pulse rate to no more than 220 minus your age

For example:

$$\frac{220 - 44 \text{ years of age}}{176 \text{ per minute}}$$

The adequate range is 120-140 beats per minute.

Chapter Three

Set Your Personal Goals

"But Daniel made up his mind that he would not defile himself with the King's choice of food or with wine ..."
(Daniel 1:8 NASB)

Setting goals is the first step to success.

Goals provide you with the focus needed to achieve what you desire and create the motivation and willpower to fulfil your objectives. The most critical factor in a diet or weight loss program is having committed goals. Studies indicate that people who write down their goals succeed in achieving them over 50 per cent more than those who don't write down goals.

Name: _____	
Commence Date: _____	
Finish Date: _____	
WEIGHT: Now: _____ Finish: _____	
WAIST: Now: _____ Finish: _____	**HIPS:** Now: _____ Finish: _____

UPPER ARMS:	THIGHS:
Now:_____ Finish:_____	Now:_____ Finish:_____

Current Health Symptoms before Starting:

_____

_____

What's most important? List your three most important goals:

_____

_____

What Could Get in My Way? List some obstacles to accomplishing your goals:

_____

_____

My Personal Scriptures/Affirmations are:

_____

_____

My Commitment Pledge

"I will commit to the diet plan and acknowledge that I may not always stick to the Plan and when that happens I won't beat myself up, rather I will get back on track with the next meal."

"I will give it 100% effort and stick to the program."

Print Name:

[   ]

Sign Name:

[   ]

The Goals of This 6-Week Healthy Eating Planner

- Give you healthy and 'Yummy' recipes
- Enhance or improve - your general health and well-being.
- To give you a working strategy that you can easily follow and enjoy.
- Show you through a good diet, exercise, a healthy lifestyle, adequate sleep, relaxation, and positive thinking, you will generate abundant physical energy and brainpower sufficient for any task, including healing and longevity.

Following this Plan will enable you to align with your goals and reduce the risk of developing many chronic diseases. You will burn fat as the body's primary fuel source and maintain or increase lean muscle mass.

What Are the Benefits for Me?

Understanding the benefits you can achieve in this 6 weeks program can be a great motivator to follow the plan.

The benefits are outstanding:
- ❖ It can change your life
- ❖ It makes your life of better quality – you enjoy life more
- ❖ You look and feel better
- ❖ Less sickness and disease

- ❖ It can improve your sex life
- ❖ Overcome cravings and sugar-related problems
- ❖ More confidence
- ❖ More energy
- ❖ Improved concentration
- ❖ More productive –you can achieve more
- ❖ You can fit into your favourite clothes again
- ❖ You can gain control over cravings back in your life.

Motivation & Help for Emotional Eating.

Avoid emotional eating. Breaking your diet because you are emotional can lead to feelings of guilt and regret making you feel worse in the end.

Changing Self Talk

Do you realize that we talk to our 'self' more in our mind than anyone else?
Therefore our self-talk must be positive, uplifting, encouraging and progressive. Stop and be aware (listen) to what you say to yourself (and others). Self-talk is all about you, what you think and what is really going on inside you, and over time it has created all your beliefs and feelings and controls what you instinctively say and do. The wonderful thing is; if it's harmful or negative, you can change it with some effort, and it's well worth it.

For example, if you are an emotional eater, the next time you feel the promptings to eat when emotionally vulnerable, stop and ask yourself – Why do I need to eat? What are you saying to yourself at that moment? Recognise it and change the self-talk.

Self-talk is key to achieving goals because it can change your internal programming. It deals directly with the root of the problem or is intimately involved with success.

Massive changes, remarkable achievements, success and happiness, can happen simply by changing one or two things in your self-talk.

If you become your own motivator, there's a greater chance of you overcoming problems, staying on a good diet and living a healthy lifestyle. Motivation means to 'put into motion.' Everyone can take control back in their life, put their decision to change into motion and follow this healthy way of living.

See yourself slimmer, trimmer and healed of all past issues. Start speaking in a way that encourages you to achieve what you want. Start telling yourself the truth - you are a wonderful, successful person who is going to accomplish all you want in life, and what's more, you're going to enjoy the journey. The most powerful motivation is your internal motivation, and now is the time to set it into motion!

Help to Stay on Track:

- Planning your meals in advance and sticking to this Plan will keep you accountable for the foods you eat and help you adhere to your program.

- Stick to a shopping list to avoid impulse purchases and purchasing foods that are not on the allowable food list. Always shop on a full stomach, and it is easier to make the right choices when you are not hungry.

- Remove as much food as practical from your home that is not on the allowable food list. Remember: "If it's in front of you, it will eventually be eaten". Called the 'See Food & Eat Food Diet'.

- ❖ Realistic expectations. A weight loss of 0.5 to 2kg a week is an achievable and maintainable goal. When setting goal weight, it is best to set small increments of weight loss and reset the next small increment when you reach that goal, etc. Also, don't weigh yourself too often – weekly to fortnightly is best.

- ❖ Ensure you have a good support network. Tell your friends and family that you are on the program, your reasons and motivations for doing it and how important your goals are to you. Try and get an exercise 'buddy'. Ask them to be supportive and not offer you junk food, as it only makes it harder for you.

- ❖ After cooking, immediately remove all excess food to avoid unnecessary and unaccounted snacking.

- ❖ If making meals in advance, split them into correct serving sizes and refrigerate or freeze them immediately.

- ❖ Drinking a large glass of water before your meal will make you feel full and help to avoid overeating. Not too close to meals as it may interfere with your digestion – (about an hour or so before is best).

- ❖ Learn to say "No" to temptation and "stop" when feeling full. Eating slowly at the table and not in front of the TV is wise. Do not have sweets and cookies in the house - Remove the temptation.

Chapter Four

The Shopping List

It's wise to know what to shop for before starting the Diet, and this avoids the risk of being caught without any of the recommended foods on hand when you are hungry, lessening the chance of being tempted back to fast food, white bread, sugar and other unhealthy foods. Air fryers are recommended as this cuts down the consumption of fried foods.

Variety of Vegetables

Alfalfa, Artichokes, Asian greens, Asparagus, Bamboo Shoots, Bean sprouts, Bok Choy,
Broccoli, Brussels sprouts, Cabbage, Capsicum, Cauliflower, Celery, Coleslaw (dry),
Cucumbers, Eggplant, Endive, Fennel, Green beans, Lettuce, Leeks, Mushrooms, Okra,
Olives, Onions, Radishes, Radicchio, Rocket, Salad greens, Sea Vegetables, Silver beets,
Shallots, Spinach, Sprouts, Squash, Tomatoes, Turnip, Watercress, Water Chestnuts, Zucchini.

Fruit. The bitter fruits are best for low GI (sugar) content. Only one piece daily would work best. You can make up for the fruit intake when doing the Daniels Diet.

Apples, Berries, Cherries, Grapefruit, Lemons, Limes, Passionfruit, Pears.

All berries- including; Blackberries, Blueberries, Mulberries, Raspberries, and Strawberries.

Nuts and Seeds

Store nuts and oils properly. Nuts and oils go sour/rancid quickly with exposure to heat, light and air. Rancid nuts smell and taste 'off' and can harm your health.

Roasted, chopped, and ground nuts go rancid much more quickly than whole raw ones. The best way to store nuts and oils is in the refrigerator, in airtight containers.

The nuts to eat on this Plan are; Almonds, Brazil nuts, Coconuts, Hazelnuts, Macadamias, Pecans, Pepitas, Pine nuts, Pistachios, Sesame seeds, Sunflower seeds, Walnuts.

Meats

Grass-fed- Beef, Lamb and Venison.

Fish and Seafood.

No farmed fish allowed. It must be ocean or wild fish only, and this goes for fish oil capsules. Fish (preferably the ones with scales, not skin, e.g. (catfish and sharks have skin).

Poultry and Eggs

Free-range Chicken, Turkey and Duck. And Eggs - including; Chicken, Duck.

Vegetable Oils

Healthy fats include coconut oil, avocado, MCT oil, butter, olive oil and raw nuts. Cold-pressed oil in dark glass bottles is the best and safest way to buy all oils. Here the liquid has been extracted without the use of chemicals or excessive heat. Light and oxygen cause rancidity, so that's why storage in dark glass is important.

Olive oil - Being a monounsaturated fat and high in oleic acid, and is one of the most stable oils and, therefore, a good choice for salads and light cooking. Organic butter is good to eat, and high-quality organic olive oil would be the best choice, with the second being extra virgin olive oil.

MCT oil is made from coconut and is a fat called Medium-chain Triglycerides (MCT) and is very good to use.

Condiments and Sauces

Tamari wheat-free Soy Sauce in moderation is OK. Curry paste (unsweetened), Coconut milk, Egg mayonnaise, Eggplant dip, Fish sauce, Horseradish, Hot pickles, Hot chilli sauce, Lemon juice, Lemon pepper, Lime juice, Mustard, Olives, Pesto, Tabasco, Tahini, Tamari, Apple cider Vinegar, Wasabi, Worcestershire sauce. Himalayan rock salt.

Herbs and Spices

- All-natural Herbs, seasonings and spices, e.g. Turmeric, Garlic, Ginger, Parsley. Organic Black Seed (Nigella seed) for my pepper taste.

Beverages

Herbal teas include; Green or Black, Rooibos, Chamomille, Peppermint, and other Herbal teas. No sugar or milk!

One or two cups of organic black coffee with one tablespoon of MCT oil added is suitable – unless you have anxiety or heart issues; if so, ask your Naturopath if it is OK. MCT oil is made from coconut and is a fat called Medium-chain Triglycerides (MCT).

Filtered water

One of the essences of good Health is to drink clean water (not tap) and to breathe clean air (air purifiers).

Dairy

If you have a dairy or lactose problem, it's best **Not** to eat any Dairy. If you have read my Diet book, you would have learnt Dairy is best avoided. Dairy foods are often allergy foods and can produce mucus. However, some people love cheese and don't have side effects from eating it. On this style of eating plan, it's OK to eat some dairy included in the recipes—your choice. If you don't want to eat dairy or any other ingredient in the recipe, that's OK just work around it by choosing the ones without it or utilise another option.

Cheeses that are very low in milk sugar (lactose) are cheddar, Parmesan (very high protein) and Swiss cheeses. As a general rule, aged cheese is low-lactose cheese, and older cheese becomes hard because it loses its moisture content and with that comes lower milk sugar; therefore, hard cheeses have much less lactose in them. Wiser choices - Cottage, Ricotta and Fetta cheese. Hard (yellow) cheese including; Colby, Cheddar, Edam, Mozzarella, Parmesan, Romano, and Swiss.

Dairy-free cheeses and milk substitutes are available. Generally, unsweetened goat milk, coconut milk, almond and hemp dairy substitutes are acceptable.

BUTTER is a high-fat product, but as such, it contains only tiny amounts of lactose. GHEE (clarified butter) is good too. Use both.

YOGURT- Goat yogurt, yes. Live cultured dairy probiotics contain relatively little lactose. Try to purchase higher-fat yogurt with live bacterial cultures.

HEAVY CREAM-The fat skimmed off the top of milk creates heavy cream, and it is about 37% fat. It contains almost no lactose (sugar), making it favourable for this diet. Therefore, unsweetened whipping cream is also OK.

SOUR CREAM-find ones, if possible, that are made from natural cream and lactose-free sour cream.

Soy Foods
Miso, Tofu and Tempeh. **No soy milk drinks**.

Sweeteners
Stevia (available at health food stores). Xylitol sugar (natural sugar found in plants). And taste like sugar and does not have the metallic taste of Stevia.

Not Allowed Food

Avoid
Gluten: Bread, Yeast based spreads, Beer, Alcohol, Pastry, Breakfast cereal, Cereal/grain coffee (chicory is OK), Gravy, Cake, Sauce, white rice, Pasta, Biscuits/Crackers, Cookies
Avoid
All sugar

Drinking chocolate, flavoured coffee chill, Sweetened coffee blends. Soft drinks, Cordials, Fruit juices, Flavoured milk.

Avoid

Table salt, but Himalayan salt is allowed. Any Sauces and condiments with added sugars, such as - Sweet Chilli, Tomato and BBQ sauce. Monosodium Glutamate (MSG), Artificial flavourings, Coloring, and Artificial preservatives. *Read the labels.*

Avoid

Polyunsaturated fats, which include common vegetable oils such as corn, soy, safflower, sunflower and canola, are not to be used in cooking. These omega-6 oils are highly susceptible to heat damage and, therefore, are not recommended at any time for general health reasons.

No margarine

Avoid

Deep-fried foods; All processed or crumbed foods. E.g. poultry such as Nuggets and Sandwich meats.

Avoid

Processed or crumbed seafood such as Nuggets, All deep fried fish and Fish fingers.

Avoid

Custard, tin fruit, Chocolate, Ice cream, Milk, Yoghurt.

Avoid

All sweetened yoghurt and soy milk. Unsweetened, and if you make your own yogurt or kefir, then that's OK to have.

Avoid

Cashews, peanuts and Salted nuts. Blue cheese and corn.

Alcohol – all

Avoid

Bananas, Grapes, Canned sweetened fruits, Dried fruits. All Fruit juices (shop bought or homemade)- because of high sugar content (high GI)

Avoid

Potatoes, Sweet Potatoes, Corn, Cassava, **White Rice.**
Corn is not a vegetable-it is a grain.
Avoid
All Sugar, Molasses, honey, fructose, and fruit concentrate. All artificial sweeteners, e.g. Aspartame

Note; if you need more detail on why not to eat certain foods and why to eat more of other specific foods, please read my book - Daniel's Diet, as I go into a lot of detail there.

Chapter Five

Intermittent Fasting (IF)

IF is optional but recommended.

From experience, I find that most people benefit from IF in many ways, which you will find out when undergoing my eating plans. But in the context of this book, it's to lose weight and regain energy.

WHAT IS INTERMITTENT FASTING - Or time-restricted feeding?

Intermittent Fasting, also called IF, is pretty easy; you eat within a short time frame of the day and don't eat (fast) the rest of the time. The good news is that there are several ways to work out what times you wish to follow so you can adapt them into your lifestyle. In other words, you can change your eating window and intermittent fasting schedule any time you want to. You can think of it as an eating schedule different from what you previously followed.

Why should you consider Intermittent Fasting?

- Intermittent Fasting can be an effective way to manage your body weight.

- There are lots of documented benefits of intermittent Fasting or time-restricted feeding. For example, it helps digestion, lowers insulin levels, causes weight loss, improves sleep (if not eating right before bed), improves blood pressure, improves cholesterol, improves brain health, and helps reduce inflammation. **And it's FREE!** All you need to do is try it and see what happens.

- One of the problems with round-the-clock picking at foods (grazing) is that your blood sugar goes up and down with what you eat. Each time it drops, you feel hungry again, even if you just ate a couple of hours ago. So we are tricked into thinking we are hungry when we are not, but it causes us to eat again, our blood sugar spikes again, then it falls again, and the whole cycle restarts. Intermittent Fasting gives your blood sugar a chance to stabilise. You should notice that you can control the cravings when you practice IF for a short time.

- Most people overeat; we don't need to eat something every few hours. Give your tummy a holiday from digesting food, as it takes enormous amounts of energy to digest and assimilate food.

There is no reason NOT to start intermittent Fasting. It may take some getting used to, but since intermittent Fasting is so flexible, you can work up to it and experiment with what suits you best.

My IF program.

I like making things as easy as possible, and this is how I do it.

1. I Skip breakfast.
2. From around 11 am, I eat my first main meal. The time never has to be exact; close enough is ok.
3. If I feel hungry before dinner, I have one piece of low GI (low sugar) fruit.
4. I eat a typical early dinner. (See the recipe section). At 7 pm.
5. **I Stop** eating by 7 pm. Best not to eat anything after this time, but you can have a cup of green or herb tea. Don't add honey or sugar.
6. Repeat this IF eating window (routine) the next day.

What I am doing on this IF timetable is not eating (fasting) between 7 pm and 11 am the next day - which is 16 hours—called the **16-hour window** for IF.

Now, if breakfast is important to you or you have doubts about this eating style because it might go against what you've previously learned, many of us were brought up being told that 'it's best not to skip a meal if you want to lose weight' –Or 'breakfast is the most important meal of the day". Rest assured; you will not starve or lack anything by following the IF system.

However, if you have misgivings about missing breakfast, there's nothing wrong with eating breakfast; you can choose to do the 16-hour window by eating breakfast and not eating dinner. You would work your second meal into the afternoon to make the 16-hour fasting time fit into the day. As I have said, you can adjust the schedule to any time that suits your lifestyle. This means shift workers, children's schedules, etc., can all undertake this IF plan by adjusting the times. Make it work for you; it will be worth the initial effort.

For example, I have breakfast with my wife once a week around 8 am as a quality time - social outing. So I simply adjust, have my next meal at 4 pm, and am still in the 16-hour window.

HOW DOES INTERMITTENT FASTING WORK?

Fasting daily and creating longer durations between meals gives your body time to reset and recover from toxic overload. When you take longer breaks between meals, your glucose levels remain stable, your insulin levels drop, and your body can clean up, eliminate harmful toxins, and lose weight.

The idea (plan) is to eat all your daily calories within a shortened period (typically a 6-8 hour window) and fast (choose not to eat) the rest of the time. This type of eating schedule is great for those who don't want to eat in the morning when they wake up. It may take a little getting used to, but try it and see what happens.

Let me encourage you and give you a few tips to help.

Tip 1. I'll drink about 1 litre (plus) of water during the course of the morning and before I eat at 11 am.
Included in that 1 litre, I drink organic green tea, and you can drink black organic coffee, too, if you wish. Use plunger coffee and not instant. I add one tablespoon of MCT oil into both of these beverages as the oil will help stop immediate food cravings and won't interfere with the fasting Detox that is taking place. If you add honey, sugar or milk of any kind, it stops the power of the fasting Detox taking place.

Tip 2. Then Some days, depending on what is happening, I'll switch it up and do 18:6 or 20:4 IF schedule. It is best to have a daily routine in place, but you do not have to be 'religious' about it; enjoy.

Tip 3. If you get hungry between meals, try snacking on keto-friendly foods. Foods that suit are hardboiled eggs, avocados, chicken leg or MCT with coffee but no more than 2 cups daily.

Tip 4. With some patients, I started them on a 12:12 schedule because they find it hard to miss a meal because of various Health or mental issues. Then when they adjust over a few weeks, I progress them up to the 14:10 window. They do this for a few weeks, then progress to the 16:8 window.

I like this eating style because it is so flexible, and you are not locked into just one rigid plan. It depends on how I feel that day, how busy I'll be in the mornings, or if I know I'm doing something with friends late at night where food will most likely be involved.

When you understand the principle of IF and want to give your body at least 12 -14 hours of not having to digest anything, you can adjust times to suit. If I eat later that evening, like 8 pm (which I avoid most times), I can start eating the next day at 1 pm, for example. I control my eating window, so there is no perceived pressure to stick to a preconceived rigid plan.

Note; IF is Not for everyone! If you are pregnant, breastfeeding, elderly, have a history of disordered eating, have an acute medical condition or are taking strong medication, speak with your healthcare practitioner about whether to engage in intermittent Fasting.

BREAKFAST RECIPES

I have included a full-day recipe so that everyone has recipe choices when you choose what window times suit you. And for those who choose not to do the IF.

1. SPINACH AND EGG BIRDS' NEST

Ingredients
- 3 handfuls spinach
- 2 tablespoons parmesan cheese, grated
- 2 eggs
- Black pepper
- 1/2 tablespoon organic butter

Method
1. Heat butter in a saucepan.
2. Wilt the spinach in a heated saucepan and squeeze the excess water out. Make into two birds' nest shapes and crack an egg into each one.
3. Sprinkle cheese and black pepper onto the top of the egg. Bake in oven at 180°C for 15 minutes or until eggs are firm. Serves 1

2. EGGS FLORENTINE

Ingredients
- 3 handfuls fresh spinach leaves
- 2 tablespoons parmesan cheese, freshly grated
- Himalayan pink salt and pepper to taste. I like using organic Black Seed (Nigella seed) for my pepper taste.
- 1 tablespoon white vinegar or try apple cider vinegar.
- 2 eggs

Method
1. Microwave spinach in a microwave-safe bowl or steam until wilted (3 to 5 minutes). Sprinkle with parmesan cheese and season to taste. Chop into bite-size pieces and place on a plate.
2. Bring the water pan to a boil, then reduce heat to a simmering point. Add vinegar and stir with a wooden spoon to create a whirl pool. Break an egg into the centre, turn off the heat and leave covered until set (3 to 4 minutes). Repeat with the second egg.

3. Place eggs on spinach and serve. Serves 1

3. KENZIE'S SALMON OMELETTE
Quick and Easy to make!

Ingredients
- 2 eggs
- 1 slice of smoked salmon
- 1/2 handful tomato, sliced
- 1 tablespoon dill, diced fresh or dried
- 1 tablespoon sour cream (low fat)
- Cracked pepper and sea salt to taste
- 1 tablespoon olive oil

Method
1. Preheat grill. Whisk eggs and dill. Add pepper and salt to taste.
2. Pour the mixture into the oiled frying pan (on medium heat) to form a thin layer. Cook for one minute in a pan and one minute under the grill.
3. Once cooked, place the omelette on a plate and lay salmon, sour cream and sliced tomato on one half of the omelette. Garnish, fill with dill and fold to form a triangle.

Serve with three handfuls of allowed vegetables or salad per serve. Serves 1

4. MEDITERRANEAN GOAT'S CHEESE AND ASPARAGUS FRITTATA

Ingredients
- 1 teaspoon extra virgin olive oil
- 2 handfuls leek, pale section only, washed, dried, thinly sliced
- 1 garlic clove, finely chopped
- 4 handfuls asparagus, woody ends trimmed, cut into 4 cm lengths
- 4 eggs
- 50 g goat's cheese, crumbled

- 1 1/2 tablespoons fresh thyme leaves
- Salt & freshly ground black pepper
- Olive oil to grease.

Method
1. Heat the oil in a medium frying pan over medium heat. Add the leek and cook, stirring, for 4 minutes or until soft. Add the garlic and cook for a further 1 minute. Remove from heat and set aside for 5 minutes to cool.
2. Meanwhile, cook the asparagus in a medium saucepan of boiling water for 3 minutes or until bright green and tender-crisp. Refresh under cold running water. Drain.
3. Using a whisk, whisk together the eggs in a large bowl until well combined. Then stir the leek mixture, asparagus, goat's cheese and thyme into it—season with salt and pepper.
4. Preheat the grill to medium to high. Heat a 23cm non-stick frying pan over medium heat. Brush the frying pan with olive oil to lightly grease. Pour the egg mixture into the prepared pan and use a spoon to smooth the mix so the asparagus and cheese are submerged. Cook for 7 minutes or until the outer edge sets.
5. Place the frying pan under the preheated grill and cook for a further 3 to 4 minutes or until golden brown and just set. Remove from grill. Set aside for 10 minutes to set. Cut frittata into wedges to serve. Serves 2

5. KRISTE'S SCRAMBLED EGGS

Ingredients
- 3 handfuls onions, mushrooms and spinach, finely chopped
- 2 eggs
- 40 g hard cheese (low fat), grated
- 2 tablespoons A2 milk
- 1 tablespoon olive oil

Method
1. Heat olive oil in a pan. Gently sauté onions, mushrooms and spinach.
2. Beat eggs, cheese and milk together, then pour into a hot pan. Stir eggs every so often till scramble appearance.
3. Serve on a plate. Serves 1

6. TURKEY SAUSAGE AND VEGETABLES

Ingredients
- 2 palm size portions of gluten-free chicken or turkey sausages
- 3 handfuls of mixed chopped onion, mushroom, tomato and green capsicum
- 3 handfuls, fresh spinach leaves, washed
- 1 tablespoon olive oil
- Cracked pepper and sea salt to taste.

Method
1. Microwave spinach in a microwave-safe bowl or steam until wilted (3 to 5 minutes). Chop into bite-size pieces and place on a plate.
2. Place chopped vegetables and sausage into a hot oiled pan and sauté until sausages are cooked through. Once sausages are cooked, chop into 1 to 2 cm slices.
3. Spoon the sausage and vegetable mixture over the spinach. Season with salt and pepper and serve. Serves 2

7. BARNY'S QUICK & EASY SMOOTHIE

Ingredients
- 1 rounded scoop of Vanilla Whey Protein shake
- 1 handful of fresh or frozen berries
- ½ an avocado
- 200 mL pure water

- Ice

Method
1. Combine ingredients and blend. Serve in a tall glass. Serves 1

8. PORRIDGE WITH PROTEIN POWDER

Ingredients
- 1/2 scoop of Vanilla Protein shake
- 1/2 palm size portion of ricotta cheese
- 1 egg
- 100 mL pure water
- Xylitol or Stevia sweetener to taste (if required)
- Vanilla essence to taste
- Cinnamon or nutmeg powder

Method
1. Mix egg, ricotta and Splenda/Stevia in a bowl. Microwave for three minutes or bake at 180°C for 20 minutes or until golden brown.
2. Blend Shake It and vanilla essence with 100 mL water to make creamy consistency and serve in a large bowl with mock porridge. Sprinkle with cinnamon or nutmeg. Serves 1

9. SCRAMBLED TOFU
Try something different

Ingredients
- 2 palm-size portions of soft/silken tofu
- 3 handfuls of diced mixed tomato, zucchini, onion or other allowed vegetables of your choice
- 1 tablespoon olive oil
- 1 teaspoon mixed herbs
- Tabasco sauce (optional)
- Cracked pepper and sea salt to taste
- Paprika to season

Method

1. Finely chop vegetables, add to the oiled frying pan and sauté with mixed herbs until tender. Add tofu, breaking up and stirring until heated through.
2. Add 2 drops of Tabasco (optional) and season with pepper and salt to taste.
3. Place on a plate and sprinkle lightly with paprika. Serve with Tabasco sauce on the side. Serves 1

10. RICOTTA AND VEGETABLE STACK

Ingredients
- 2 large flat-field mushrooms
- 2 handfuls of mixed eggplant, capsicum and zucchini
- Sun-dried tomato pesto
- 1 tablespoon fresh chives, chopped
- 2 tablespoons toasted pine nuts
- 1 teaspoon crushed garlic
- 1 teaspoon lemon rind, finely grated
- 1 palm size portion of ricotta cheese
- 1 tablespoon olive oil

Method
1. Cut eggplant, zucchini and capsicum into strips, leave mushrooms whole and grill or fry with olive oil until tender.
2. Combine ricotta, chives, garlic and lemon rind in a bowl.
3. Place cooked mushrooms stem side up on a plate and layer with cheese mixture and slices of eggplant, capsicum and zucchini. Dress generously with pesto and sprinkle with pine nuts. Serves 1

11. YUMMY SALMON BREAKFAST
With leftover roast vegetables...

Ingredients
- 2 handfuls of leftover or freshly baked vegetables, e.g. zucchini, capsicum, eggplant
- 1 handful of rocket leaves
- 1 palm size portion of smoked salmon

- 2 teaspoons lemon juice
- 1 teaspoon olive oil
- Cracked pepper and sea salt to taste.

Method
1. Sauté leftover vegetables in an oiled frying pan to heat.
2. Serve hot vegetables with salmon and rocket. Drizzle with lemon juice and add cracked pepper to taste. Serves 1

12. STRAWBERRY AND SILKEN TOFU SMOOTHIE
Try this unusual Smoothie!

Ingredients
- 1 handful strawberries
- 1 palm size portion of silken tofu
- 350 ml A2 milk
- Stevia sweetener to taste
- Cinnamon (optional)

Method
1. Combine silken tofu, milk and strawberries in a blender and blend until smooth.
2. Add sweetener to taste. Sprinkle with cinnamon (optional) and serve in a tall glass. Serves 1

13. VANILLA PROTEIN PANCAKES
What? A healthy pancake?

Ingredients
- 1 scoop of Vanilla Protein Shake
- 1 tablespoon of almond or hazelnut meal
- 30 mL water
- 1 egg

Method
1. Combine ingredients in a bowl.

2. In a non-stick pan, cook on moderate heat for approx 2 to 3 minutes on each side. You can use olive oil or a small amount of butter to prevent sticking. Observe as it may burn quickly.
3. Try serving buttered with a handful of mixed berries or stewed apple and cinnamon. Serves 1 (4 pancakes)

14. SCRAMBLED EGGS – WITH FRUIT

Ingredients
- 2 eggs
- 50 ml A2 milk
- 1 handful of your choice of allowed low-carbohydrate fruits
- Cinnamon (optional)

Method
1. Place your choice of fruits in a bowl and sprinkle with cinnamon. Set aside.
2. Whisk eggs in a bowl with a dash of milk. Pour mixture into a hot, oiled fry pan. Stir intermittently to keep eggs fluffy. Once eggs are cooked through, remove from pan and serve with fruits.
3. Eggs may be seasoned with cinnamon, sea salt, paprika, Tabasco, or pepper.
4. Serve with 3 handfuls of allowed vegetables or salad per serve. Serves 1

15. MUSHROOM FRITTATA

Ingredients
- 4 large flat mushrooms, sliced
- 1 onion, diced
- 1 clove garlic, crushed
- 2 handfuls baby spinach, washed
- 12 pitted green olives, chopped
- 4 tablespoons ricotta cheese or feta cheese
- 8 eggs
- 1 teaspoon butter

- 2 teaspoons olive oil
- Salt and pepper to taste

Method
1. Heat mushrooms, garlic, one teaspoon of olive oil, butter, salt and pepper in a covered frying pan for a few minutes until mushrooms begin to soften. Remove lid and allow to sauté until tender. Remove from pan and set aside.
2. Sauté onions in a frying pan in 1 teaspoon of olive oil until tender. Add baby spinach and toss over low heat until wilted.
3. Combine spinach, onion, olives and mushrooms and mix well.
4. Whisk the eggs and ricotta with salt and pepper in a separate bowl until the eggs are aerated. There should be pieces of ricotta remaining throughout the egg mixture.
5. In a non-stick oven pan, place the vegetable mixture evenly across the base. Pour over the egg mixture to cover.
6. Cooking times will vary, depending on the depth of the tray used - the frittata should be 3 to 6 cm high. Bake at 160°C for 20 to 30 minutes or until set.
7. Serve with 1 ½ additional handfuls of allowed vegetables or salad per serve. Serves 3

16. SPANISH-STYLE OMELETTE

Ingredients
- 2 eggs
- 1 tablespoon pure water
- Cayenne or black pepper
- 3 handfuls of finely chopped vegetables, e.g. olives, onions, chives, capsicum, parsley, spinach, and zucchini.
- 1 tablespoon of olive oil

Method

1. Lightly stir-fry vegetables in extra virgin olive oil and remove to one side.
2. Lightly mix eggs with one tablespoon of water and a pinch of pepper and pour the mixture into a heated frying pan so it covers the base of the pan. When almost cooked, place vegetables on top of half the omelette. Lift one side of the omelette over to enclose the filling.
3. Flip to heat the omelette through. Serves 1

17. SCRAMBLED SILKEN TOFU
A 'Yummy' vegetarian protein breakfast.

Ingredients
- 2 palm-size portions of soft/silken tofu
- 25 ml milk (you can try almond milk - unsweetened, malt-free) or water
- 1/2 handful of fresh herbs, e.g. basil, parsley, coriander
- 1 dessertspoon olive oil
- Cracked pepper and sea salt to taste

Method
1. Break up tofu in a bowl with a fork and add a dash of milk or water. Whisk.
2. In another bowl, toss fresh herbs with one dessert spoon of olive oil.
3. Add tofu mixture into a hot oiled frying pan. Stir often to ensure a desirable consistency.
4. When slightly browned, fold in oil-infused fresh herbs.
5. Season with sea salt and cracked black pepper if needed.
6. Serve with three handfuls of allowed vegetables or salad per serve. Serves 1

18. Protein Pan Fry

Ingredients
- Your choice of a palm size portion of meat, e.g. beef, lamb, or chicken
- 3 handfuls of diced vegetables, e.g. capsicum, mushroom, onion, zucchini, tomato
- 1 tablespoon olive oil
- Cracked pepper and sea salt to taste

Method
1. Place a selection of meat and vegetables in an oiled pan or grill. Fry or grill until cooked and serve.
2. Add cracked pepper to taste. Serves 1

19. HEALTHY VEGETABLE FRITTATA
makes an excellent cold lunch or snack!

Ingredients
- 6 handfuls of coarsely chopped vegetables, e.g. zucchini, red capsicum, broccoli, shallots and carrot
- 100 g fetta, crumbled
- 6 eggs
- 1 tablespoon olive oil
- 1/2 handful mixed fresh herbs, finely chopped, e.g. basil, parsley, chives, oregano

Method
1. Coarsely cut and steam vegetables until tender; set aside. Whisk eggs and herbs.
2. Add oil to a thick base frying pan and place on a very low heat. Add half of the egg mixture to the pan and cook for one minute.
3. Place vegetables and crumbled fetta in a pan and cover with the remaining egg mixture. Cover with a lid and cook on very low heat until cooked through.
4. Place the uncovered frying pan under the grill until the top of the frittata turns golden brown. Serves 2

20. ZUCCHINI FRITTERS
An excellent substitute for hash browns

Ingredients
- 3 handfuls grated zucchini
- 2 eggs
- 1 tablespoon olive oil for cooking
- Sprinkle of nutmeg (optional)
- Cracked pepper and sea salt to taste
- ½ size piece of salmon

Method
1. Combine all ingredients, except olive oil, in a medium bowl. Stir until well combined.
2. Heat oil in a large pan over medium to high heat. Mould the mixture into medium size balls and press flat into the pan. When brown on one side, turn and cook on the other side.
3. Serve with ½ size piece of salmon. Serves 1

21. Stuffed Mushroom & Cheese

Ingredients
- Field Mushrooms (big)x2
- Feta Cheese 100g (grated)
- Ricotta Cheese (firm) 200g
- 3 Eggs
- 1 tbsp parsley
- ½ cup grated zucchini
- ½ baby spinach
- 1 tbsp chopped onion

Method
1. Lightly fry chopped onions in olive oil.
2. Add baby spinach, mushrooms and zucchini to the pan and lightly fry.
3. In a bowl, mix grated feta cheese, ricotta and egg.
4. Add cooked ingredients from the pan to the bowl, and add parsley mix.

5. Spoon mixture evenly onto mushrooms and bake in the oven at 180 degrees Celsius for approximately 30 minutes or until lightly browned. Serves 2

Snacks RECIPES

1. MUNG BEAN SNACK MIX

Ingredients
- 3 handfuls of mung bean sprouts
- 1 1/2 handfuls lentil sprouts
- 1 1/2 handfuls sunflower seed sprouts
- 1 handful of chickpea sprouts
- 1 handful of clover sprouts
- 1 handful of radish sprouts
- 2 teaspoons thyme leaves
- 2 teaspoons oregano
- 1 teaspoon marjoram leaves
- 1/2 teaspoon rosemary
- 1 teaspoon garlic powder
- 1 teaspoon tamari (wheat-free soy sauce)
- 1 teaspoon extra virgin olive oil

Method
1. Mix sprouts together in a large bowl.
2. Mix herbs, garlic powder and tamari together in a small jar.
3. Sprinkle one tablespoon of herb seasoning over the sprouts in a bowl. Store any remaining herb seasoning in a capped jar for another use.
4. Drizzle sprout mixture with olive oil and toss to mix. Serve immediately.
5. It can be used per handful as a side dish or added to salad. Serves 3 (Vegetable Side Dish)

2. SAVOURY AND SPICY NUTS

Ingredients
- 1 tablespoon butter
- 1/3 cup tamari soy sauce
- 2 teaspoons ground ginger powder
- 1/4 teaspoon wasabi paste (optional)
- 2 cups walnuts
- 1 cup almonds or pecans
- 1 cup raw Brazil or hazelnuts

Method
1. Preheat oven to 150°C.
2. Melt butter in a small saucepan over low heat.
3. Combine soy sauce, ginger and wasabi paste in a small bowl.
4. Spread nuts over a baking tray.
5. Pour on butter and stir to coat.
6. Bake for about 15 minutes.
7. Remove from oven. Stir in the ginger-soy mixture.
8. Return to oven and roast for about 10 minutes more.
9. Let stand at room temperature to cool. Store in an airtight container. Serves 12 (Snack)

3. TURKEY MINCE IN LETTUCE CUPS

Ingredients
- 2 palm size portions of TURKEY mince
- 1 cup sliced water chestnuts, drained
- 1 tablespoon sliced ginger
- 1 tablespoon chilli sauce
- 1 tablespoon tamari wheat-free soy sauce
- Iceberg lettuce leaves, cut carefully into cups

Method
Sauté ginger lightly before browning turkey mince. Add sauces with water chestnuts and simmer for five minutes. Thin with a bit of water. Spoon mixture into lettuce cups for serving. Serves 4 (Snack)

4 JESSA'S QUICHE
Excellent served cold as a snack

Ingredients
- 4 eggs
- 1 finely sliced medium onion
- 1/2 handful zucchini, grated
- 1/2 handful broccoli, finely chopped
- 40 g hard cheese (low fat), grated

Method
1. Combine all ingredients together and spoon into a quiche dish. Bake in a moderate oven for 25 minutes until the quiche is set. Serves 4 (Snack)

6. ROCKET AND PEAR SALAD WITH BLUE CHEESE DRESSING

Ingredients
- 2 handfuls of baby rocket leaves
- 1 handful of thinly sliced pear, skin on
- 1/4 cup roasted walnuts, chopped
- 3 tablespoons white wine vinegar
- 4 tablespoons extra virgin olive oil
- 2 teaspoons Dijon mustard
- 1 tablespoon lemon juice
- 1 tablespoon blue cheese
- Pinch of salt
- Pinch of pepper

Method
1. To make dressing blend the last seven ingredients or whisk together thoroughly.
2. Place rocket leaves pear, walnuts, and half the dressing in a large bowl and combine lightly.
3. Transfer to a serving dish and drizzle over more dressing if required. Serves 1 (Vegetable Side Dish)

7. SPINACH AND CHICKEN STUFFED MUSHROOMS

Ingredients
- 1 handful spinach
- 1 palm size portion of chicken breast, finely diced
- 4 medium mushrooms
- 1 teaspoon butter
- 1 clove garlic
- 1 teaspoon oregano
- 1 teaspoon lemon juice
- 3 tablespoons cheese (low fat), grated

Method
1. Preheat oven to 200°C and grease tray. Wash spinach and place in a lightly oiled saucepan (no water added) on moderate heat until spinach wilts. Drain and cool spinach and squeeze out excess liquid.
2. Chop stems off mushrooms and keep. Melt butter in a saucepan. Add garlic, herbs, chicken, and mushroom stems and cook until golden.
3. Mix in spinach and cook for 1 minute. Stir in lemon juice and remove from heat.
4. Fill mushroom caps with mixture and sprinkle with cheese—place in the oven for 10 to 15 minutes or until cheese has melted. Serves 2 (Snack)

7. SOY AND GARLIC KEBABS
Served cold, this is the ultimat ready to eat fat loss snack

Ingredients
- 1 palm size portion of chicken breast, cut into cubes
- 1 1/2 handfuls onion and green capsicum, cut into wedges
- 1 1/2 handfuls cherry tomatoes
- 2 tablespoons garlic, crushed
- Chilli paste (optional)
- 3 tablespoons soy sauce
- Pinch salt

- Cracked black pepper
- Wooden skewers

Method
1. Soak wooden skewers in water for ½ hour so they do not burn.
2. Pierce the chicken and vegetables onto the skewers. Mix garlic, soy and seasoning in a small bowl and brush kebabs with the mixture.
3. Cook in a pan, BBQ or under the grill until chicken is cooked through. Serves 2 (Snack)

8. CAULIFLOWER RICE SUBSTITUTE
This dish is a great rice substitute

Ingredients
- 3 handfuls cauliflower, grated
- 1 tablespoon olive oil

Method
1. Grate the cauliflower using the medium-sized holes of a grater. Grate the core too. With your hands, squeeze out as much water as you can. This may not be necessary for some cauliflower as they vary in degree of wetness.
2. Add the grated cauliflower to a heated and oiled wok or pan and fry until it's tender-crisp, about 5 to 8 minutes. The length of time will depend on the cauliflower.
3. Use as you would rice. The variations are endless. Serves 1 (Vegetable Side Dish)

9. BLUEBERRY AND RICOTTA CREPES
Delicious served hot

Ingredients
- 1 large egg
- 1 tablespoon cream
- 1 teaspoon oil
- 1/4 teaspoon Splenda

- 3 drops vanilla essence
- 100 g ricotta
- 1 handful of fresh blueberries

Method
1. Mix egg, cream, Splenda and vanilla essence in a bowl. Put in a well-buttered non-stick frying pan and swirl to coat the pan.
2. Cook at medium to high heat until the top looks dry; flip over and cook for a few more seconds. Place on a plate and fill with ricotta and blueberries. Ricotta can be sweetened with Splenda. Serves 2

10. LEMON CAKE

Ingredients
- 1 1/3 cups almond meal
- 4 teaspoons xilitol
- 4 eggs separated
- 5 teaspoons grated lemon peel
- 1/2 teaspoon ground cinnamon
- Pinch of salt

Method
1. Preheat oven to 180°C. Butter and flour a 9-inch diameter cake pan with 1 1/2-inch high sides. Line the bottom of the pan with waxed paper.
2. Combine yolks, add Stevia to taste, lemon peel, cinnamon and salt in a medium bowl. Using an electric mixer, beat until thick and smooth (approximately 2 minutes). Stir in almond meal and two more teaspoons of Splenda.
3. Using clean beaters, beat egg whites in a large bowl until soft peaks form. Gradually add four teaspoons of Splenda, beating until stiff but not dry. Fold a large spoonful of whites into the almond mixture. Gently fold in the remaining whites.

4. Transfer the batter to the pan. Bake until the skewer comes out clean (approximately 35 minutes). Cool in pan on rack. Turn out onto a platter. Remove waxed paper. Cut into six slices. Serves 6 (Snack)

11. COTTAGE CHEESE AND CELERY STICKS
Suitable for the lunch box

Ingredients
- 60 g cottage cheese (low fat)
- 1/2 palm size portion of tuna, tinned in brine or spring water
- 2 large celery sticks, stringed
- 3 teaspoons nut meal
- 1 tablespoon chives
- 1 tablespoon parsley

Method
1. Trim celery sticks. Mix cheese with strained tuna, parsley and chives.
2. Fill the cavity of celery sticks with the mixture. Sprinkle nut meal on top and press into filling.
3. Cut sticks into small lengths and serve. Serves 2 (Snack)

12. Guacamole

Ingredients
- 3 ripe avocados, pitted, skinned, and mashed
- Juice of 1 organic lemon
- 2 Tbsp. organic apple cider vinegar
- 1/2 cup organic coconut milk
- Fresh or ground dill and/or cilantro (oregano is great as well)
- Pink salt (Himalayan Salt) for flavor
- Serve with cucumbers, red cabbage, celery, etc.

Method

1. In a large bowl, mix together the avocados, coconut milk, lemon juice, and vinegar until well combined. Stir in the herbs and salt until the mixture is fully combined.

2. Serve with cucumbers, red cabbage, celery, bell peppers or other veggies or flax seed crackers.

Chapter Six

LUNCHES / DINNER

VEGETARIAN

1. MISO SOUP WITH TOFU
Served with veggies

Ingredients
- 1 teaspoon miso paste
- 500 mL vegetable stock
- 1 handful of shallots, chopped
- 6 cm stick Kombu or Wakame, cut into thin strips with scissors
- 2 palm-size portions of firm tofu
- 1 tablespoon tahini
- 1 tablespoon lemon juice
- 2 teaspoons soy sauce or tamari (wheat-free soy sauce)

Method
1. Add vegetable stock and kombu in a large saucepan and simmer until the kombu expands.
2. Add tofu and shallots and simmer for 5 minutes.
3. Mix in miso paste, and let come to a simmer (do not overheat), then remove from heat.
4. Mix tahini, lemon juice, tamari, and one tablespoon of water in a jar.
5. Serve Miso soup in bowls, then mix in 1 tablespoon of tahini.
6. Serve with three handfuls of vegetables such as broccoli, green beans and/or bok choy. Serves 1

2. TOFU AND BOK CHOY- with Asian flavour

Ingredients
- 6 handfuls bok choy
- 4 palm-size portions of firm tofu
- 3/4 cup vegetable stock
- 1 teaspoon butter (optional)
- 12 drops of sesame oil
- Pinch of Chinese five spice
- Soy sauce to taste

Method
1. Wash bok choy and trim ends. Cut off the leaf portion and keep it whole. Slice stems.
2. Slice tofu into strips.
3. Heat stock in a pan and add bok choy stems and tofu. Stir regularly over heat until stems are tender. Add leaves, soy sauce, sesame oil, butter and five spice and cook for another minute or until leaves soften.
4. Serve with any remaining broth. Serves 2

3. TEMPEH WITH AVOCADO, SUN-DRIED TOMATO AND MACADAMIA DIPS

Ingredients
- 1 tablespoon olive oil
- 4 palm-size portions of tempeh, cut into thin fingers
- 2 tablespoons sundried tomatoes, diced
- 1 tablespoon roasted macadamias, chopped
- 1 tablespoon fresh basil, chopped
- 1 avocado
- 1 chilli, deseeded and chopped
- 1 spring onion, chopped
- 1 tablespoon Spanish onion, chopped
- Squeeze of lemon
- 1 teaspoon sea salt

- Ground black pepper to taste

Method
1. Pan-fry the tempeh fingers in olive oil until golden and crispy.
2. Blend sundried tomatoes, macadamias, basil and pepper to the consistency of a chunky dip.
3. Mash avocado and add chilli, spring onion, Spanish onion, lemon juice, salt and pepper and mix well into a dip.
4. Arrange equal servings of tempeh fingers per person and serve with a dollop of each dip.
5. Serve with three additional handfuls of allowed vegetables or salad per serve. Serves 2

4. TEMPEH AND CAULIFLOWER CURRY

Ingredients
- 6 palm-size portions of tempeh, cut into 2 cm cubes
- 2 tablespoons olive oil
- 1/2 handful onion, chopped
- 2 medium garlic cloves
- 1 1/2 handfuls broccoli
- 1 1/2 handfuls snow peas
- 3 handfuls cauliflower
- 1 1/2 handfuls zucchini, diced
- 1 handful of mushrooms, sliced
- 2 tablespoons curry powder
- 1/2 teaspoon ground cinnamon
- 2 mild green chillies, seeded and chopped
- 1 can coconut milk (low fat)
- 1/2 cup toasted sesame seeds
- 1 tablespoon soy sauce or tamari (wheat-free soy sauce)
- Coriander, chopped to garnish

Method
1. Heat a large frying pan over medium-high. Add one tablespoon olive oil, onions, garlic and sauté until onions are translucent.

2. Add broccoli, cauliflower, snow peas, and diced zucchini, and cook for a few minutes.
3. Add curry, cinnamon, chillies, and coconut milk, stirring to combine.
4. Cover and simmer for 10 minutes (until you have finished browning tempeh in the next step).
5. In a small frying pan, heat one tablespoon olive oil, add tempeh pieces and sauté, stirring frequently, over medium heat, until tempeh pieces are golden. Remove from heat and splash with tamari soy sauce.
6. Add the tempeh to the curried vegetables and stir to combine.
7. Sprinkle with sesame seeds and coriander. Serve immediately. Serves 3

5. CURRIED TOFU

Ingredients
- 2 palm-size portions of firm tofu, diced
- 1 tablespoon extra virgin olive oil
- 1/2 handful onion, diced
- 1/2 handful celery, diced
- 1 handful of capsicum, diced
- 1 handful of green beans, diced
- 1 clove garlic, crushed
- 1/2 to 1 teaspoon curry powder
- 1 cup chicken stock
- Ground pepper and sea salt to taste

Method
1. Heat oil in a frying pan and sauté onion, garlic, celery, capsicum and green beans for approximately 3 minutes.
2. Add tofu and stir into the pan with curry powder. Add salt and pepper.
3. Add stock to the pan, bring to a boil and simmer until stock reduces. Stir occasionally. Serves 1

Salad Bar

1. CHICKEN COLESLAW

Ingredients
- 1 palm size portion of chicken breast, steamed and finely sliced
- 3 handfuls cabbage, carrot, and red onion, finely chopped
- 1/4 cup chopped parsley, chives
- 2 tablespoons crushed walnuts
- 2 tablespoons mayonnaise (whole egg, no added sugar)

Method
1. Combine all ingredients in a bowl, mix thoroughly and serve. Serves 1

2. KOREAN CHICKEN SALAD

Ingredients
- 2 palm-size portions of chicken breast

Marinade
- 2 tablespoons soy sauce
- 1 tablespoon olive oil
- 1/4 teaspoon ground ginger
- 1/4 teaspoon cinnamon
- 1 clove garlic, finely chopped

Salad
- 2 handfuls lettuce, shredded
- 1 handful cucumber, thinly sliced
- 1 handful of capsicum, thinly sliced
- 1/2 handful red onion, chopped
- 1/2 handful of snow peas
- 1 handful of bean sprouts
- 1 tablespoon slivered almonds, toasted and salted
- 1 tablespoon sesame seeds, toasted

Dressing
- 1/2 teaspoon dry mustard

- 1/2 teaspoon salt
- 1/2 teaspoon Tabasco sauce
- 1 tablespoon soy sauce
- 1 tablespoon sesame oil
- 4 teaspoons lemon juice

Method
1. Cut chicken breast in half.
2. Combine marinade ingredients and thoroughly coat chicken pieces.
3. Place chicken in a shallow roasting pan, pour the remainder of the marinade over the top and cook uncovered at 200°C for 15 to 20 minutes, turning at half time.
4. Cool the cooked chicken and cut it into thin strips.
5. Prepare salad vegetables and place in a large bowl.
6. Combine dressing ingredients and just before serving toss the chicken, salad and dressing with sesame seeds and slivered almonds.
Serves 2

3. MEDITERRANEAN SALAD

Ingredients
- 2 handfuls of salad greens - include bitter greens such as rocket or watercress
- 1 egg, hardboiled and sliced
- 1 handful mixed red onion and cucumber, sliced
- 1/2 palm size portion of tuna, tinned in brine or spring water
- 4 black olives (optional)
- 1 tablespoon extra virgin olive oil
- 1 tablespoon lemon juice or vinegar (apple cider, red wine or balsamic)

<u>Optional extras to add variety</u>: Blanched green beans, asparagus, oven-roasted capsicum or eggplant strips, and marinated mushrooms. (Use one handful to replace one handful of greens)

Method
1. Dressing: toss salad with extra virgin olive oil and sprinkle with vinegar or lemon juice.
Serves 1

4. HORROCKS BEACH TUNA SALAD
A protein-rich salad

Ingredients
- 1/2 palm size portion of tuna, tinned in brine or spring water
- 1 egg
- 3 handfuls of mixed shredded lettuce, celery, shallots, parsley, and thinly sliced fresh mushrooms
- 1 teaspoon sesame seeds
- 1 tablespoon fresh herbs
- Juice of 1 lemon
- Ground pepper to taste
- Olive oil

Method
1. Shallow fry sesame seeds until lightly browned; put aside to cool.
2. Add olive oil to a non-stick frying pan. Break up tuna in a small mixing bowl. Mix with raw egg and black pepper. Cook tuna mix over moderate heat for 8 to 10 minutes. Stir frequently, breaking up larger clumps until light golden brown and flaky. Set aside to cool.
3. Add salad and vegetables to the salad bowl. Drizzle with olive oil, add lemon juice and fresh herbs. Gently toss the cooled flaky tuna and egg mixture into a salad and sprinkle with toasted sesame seeds.
Serves 1.

4. NORTHAMPTON FRESH CHICKEN SALAD

Ingredients
- 2 palm-size portions of chicken breast, steamed and finely sliced

- 1 handful of celery, sliced
- 1 handful of red capsicum, sliced
- 1 handful of snow peas
- 2 handfuls lettuce
- 1 handful avocado, sliced
- 1 handful of tomato cut into wedges
- A squeezed lemon
- Cracked black pepper
- 1 tablespoon olive oil

Method
1. Combine all ingredients together, dress with lemon juice, pepper and olive oil. Serve immediately. Serves 2

6. KALBARI PRAWN SALAD
Seafood salad

Ingredients
- 1/2 handful avocado, sliced
- 3 handfuls of mixed salad greens
- 1 palm size portion of king prawns (approximately six prawns), cooked and peeled
- Juice of 1/2 a lime

Method
1. Cover a plate of greens with prawns. Garnish with thin slices of avocado. Dress with lime juice. Serves 1

7. SALMON NICOISE

Ingredients
- 1 palm size portion of red salmon, tinned in brine or spring water, drained and chunked
- 2 eggs, hardboiled and cut into quarters
- 2 handfuls romaine lettuce, leaves torn
- 1 1/2 handfuls artichoke hearts, drained and quartered
- 8 black and green olives

- 1 handful cucumber or zucchini, shredded or julienne
- 1 1/2 handfuls broccoli sprouts
- 1/2 handful of small sweet capsicum
- 1/2 handful avocado, peeled and cut into cubes
- 1/2 teaspoon Dijonnaise Sauce
- Lemon wedges, garnish

Method
1. Arrange lettuce on a large serving platter. Arrange mounds of the other ingredients over the platter.
2. Spritz with a splash of lemon juice.
3. Serve immediately with a small bowl of Dijonnaise Sauce. Serves 2

Fish and Seafood

1. BAKED WHITE FISH & TOASTED ALMONDS

Ingredients
- 2 palm size portions of white fish
- 2 handfuls each of green beans, broccoli florets, zucchini
- 1/2 handful of onions, thinly sliced
- 3/4 cup vegetable stock
- 1 tablespoon fresh parsley, chopped
- 1 small clove garlic, crushed
- 1 teaspoon almonds, slivered, toasted
- 1 tablespoon fresh marjoram
- 1 tablespoon olive oil
- Sea salt

Method
1. Clean, wash and dry fish.
2. Coat a shallow casserole dish with olive oil. Add garlic, onions and fry gently until onions are soft and golden. Place the fish on top of the onion mixture, pour over vegetable stock, then sprinkle with parsley, marjoram and sea salt.

3. Bake in preheated oven at 200ºC until cooked (up to 25 minutes); baste a few times.
4. Steam green vegetables till tender and strain. In a frying pan, lightly toast slivered almonds until golden and put aside to cool.
5. Serve fish with garnished toasted slivered almonds and green vegetables. Serves 2

2. WHITE FISH TAJINE

Ingredients
- 4 palm-size portions of white fish, cut into 2 cm pieces
- 2 palm-size portions of calamari tubes, cleaned and sliced
- 2 palm-size portions of king prawns (approximately 10 to 12 prawns), peeled and deveined

Marinade
- 1/2 tablespoon olive oil
- 1 tablespoon crushed garlic
- Juice of 1/2 lime (or lemon)
- Salt and pepper to taste
- 1 teaspoon ground cumin
- 1/2 cup fresh coriander, chopped roughly

Sauce
- 1 handful of roasted red capsicum, peeled
- 2 handfuls fresh tomatoes
- 1 1/2 handfuls celery, chopped
- 1 teaspoon ground cumin
- 1 tablespoon tomato paste (no added sugar)
- A small handful of fresh coriander leaves
- Salt and pepper to taste

Method
1. In a mixing bowl, combine the ingredients for the marinade and mix well.
2. Add the fish pieces, calamari and prawns. Mix so the seafood is well coated and marinate for 4 hours.
3. To make the sauce, blend the tomatoes, capsicum, including the seeds, celery and cumin.

4. Heat 1 teaspoon olive oil on high heat in a large frying pan and fry the red onion until soft. Add the blended sauce mixture and bring to a high simmer. Stir in the tomato paste, salt, pepper, coriander leaves and little cumin.
5. Cover the base of the tajine with some of the sauce, add the seafood, and then cover the seafood with the remaining sauce. Place the tajine plate on the stove over medium heat for a few minutes to start cooking. Then transfer to the oven, preheated at 180°C for 40 to 45 mins.
6. Serve with two additional handfuls of allowed vegetables or salad per serve. Serves 4

3. SEA BASS WITH CURRY SAUCE

Ingredients
- 1 palm size portion of seabass or white fish
- 4 teaspoons soy sauce
- 1 tablespoon lime juice
- 1 tablespoon lemongrass, sliced
- 1 kaffir lime leaf
- 2 to 4 red chillies, deseeded
- 1 tablespoon fresh coriander, finely chopped
- 2 tablespoons fresh basil, finely chopped
- 1 tablespoon red curry paste (no added sugar)
- 50 mL coconut milk (low fat)
- 100 mL vegetable stock
- 3 handfuls bok choy
- Ground pepper and sea salt to taste

Method
1. Preheat oven to 180°C
2. Finely chop the lemongrass, kaffir lime, red chilli and coriander leaf.
3. Mix together half of the herbs with two teaspoons of soy sauce and lime juice.
4. Marinate fish fillets on both sides in this mixture for 20 minutes.

5. Place fish on aluminium foil and basil leaves on top of fish.
6. Fold foil around fish, place in oven and cook for 15 to 20 minutes or until fish is cooked through.
7. Blanch bok choy slightly in hot water, and remove from water.
8. Lightly sauté bok choy with one teaspoon of soy sauce.
9. Sauté the remaining mixture of herbs with coconut milk until fragrant. Add red curry paste and stir until dissolved. Add coconut milk and vegetable stock, boil, and simmer until the sauce is thick but runny—season with salt and pepper.
10. Remove from heat: Place baked fish fillets on a bed of sautéed bok choy and spoon over curry sauce. Serves 1

4. NUT-CRUSTED FISH

Ingredients
- 2 tablespoons extra virgin olive oil
- 2 tablespoons butter
- 1/3 cup nuts, finely chopped
- 1 teaspoon Celtic sea salt
- Black pepper to taste
- 2 palm size portions of boneless fish
- 2 teaspoons fresh chopped parsley (optional)
- 6 handfuls salad greens
- 1 lemon

Method
1. Preheat oven to 220°C. Grease a baking sheet. Melt olive oil and butter in a pan. Remove from heat and let cool. Mix the chopped nuts together with the seasoning and put on a plate.
2. Dip the fish in the oil/butter mixture and then the nut mixture; press firmly so the nuts hold. Place fish on the baking sheet and bake until cooked through.
3. Garnish with fresh parsley. Serve with salad greens and a wedge of lemon. Serves 2

5. NOVA'S POACHED SALMON

Ingredients
- 1/4 cup lemon juice
- 1 teaspoon sea salt
- 4 palm size portions of salmon fillets
- 1 tablespoon Dijonnaise sauce

Method
1. Pour 3 to 4 cm deep of water, lemon juice, and salt into a large, deep ceramic casserole or fish poacher and bring to a boil. Reduce heat to simmer.
2. Place salmon fillets into simmering water and poach gently for 5 to 8 minutes.
3. Remove to serving dish or platter. Serve topped with or accompanied by Dijonnaise Sauce.
4. Serve with three handfuls per serve of allowed vegetables or salad. Serves 4

6. TUNA DISH
For the lunch box

Ingredients
- 60 g cottage cheese (low fat)
- 1/2 palm size portion of tuna, tinned in brine or spring water
- 2 large celery sticks, stringed
- 3 teaspoons nut meal
- 1 tablespoon chives
- 1 tablespoon parsley

Method
1. Trim celery sticks. Mix cheese with strained tuna, parsley and chives.
2. Fill the cavity of celery sticks with the mixture. Sprinkle nut meal on top and press into filling.
3. Cut sticks into small lengths and serve. Serves 2 (Snack)

7. ANNES CURRY PRAWNS

Ingredients
- 2 palm-size portions of king prawns (approximately 10 to 12 prawns) cooked, peeled and deveined
- 2 palm-size portions of firm tofu, sliced into 1 cm strips
- 250 mL coconut cream (low fat)
- 1-litre water
- 1 tablespoon fish sauce
- 1/2 teaspoon salt
- 2 teaspoons xylitol or Stevia (optional)
- 3 handfuls button mushrooms, chopped
- 3 handfuls of snow peas
- Juice 1/2 lime to taste
- A few sprigs of coriander leaves and stem, roughly chopped
- 3 handfuls of bean sprouts

Laksa paste
- 3 long red chillies, deseeded and chopped
- 1 onion, chopped
- 2 garlic cloves, chopped
- 1 lemongrass stem, white part only, finely chopped
- 1 tablespoon sesame oil
- 1/2 teaspoon shrimp paste
- 2 tablespoons mild/medium curry powder
- 1/2 teaspoon ground turmeric
- 1/4 teaspoon ground cloves

Method
1. To make the laksa paste, combine chilli, onion, garlic, lemongrass and sesame oil in a food processor and blend into a smooth paste. Heat 1 to 2 tablespoons of water in a saucepan, add the paste and stir-fry for about 2 minutes, stirring constantly until fragrant. Add the remaining paste ingredients and stir-fry for a further 1 to 2 minutes.

2. Add the coconut cream, water, tofu, fish sauce, salt and Splenda/Stevia (optional), and bring to the boil. Add snow peas, mushrooms and prawns, and simmer for a few minutes until vegetables are tender.
3. Turn off the heat and add lime juice, coriander and bean sprouts. Check for seasoning and adjust with salt or lime juice as needed. Ladle into bowls and serve. Serves 3

8. GRILLED SALMON WITH DILL BUTTER

Ingredients
- 2 palm-size portions of salmon fillets
- 2 tablespoons extra virgin olive oil
- 3 handfuls of rocket leaves (or mescalin mix)
- 1 handful of red capsicum, thinly sliced
- 1 handful of snow peas
- 1 handful of green beans

Dill butter sauce
- 60 grams of organic butter
- Juice from ½ a freshly squeezed lemon
- 2 tablespoons dried or chopped fresh dill

Method
1. Lightly steam green beans, snow peas and capsicum, set aside.
2. Brush both sides of the salmon with olive oil and grill under high heat for 3 to 4 minutes per side. Salmon is cooked when the meat is just starting to fall apart.
3. To make the sauce: Melt the butter in a small saucepan, stir in the lemon juice and add dill. Spread rocket on a dinner plate, place salmon on top and cover with warm sauce.
4. Serve with steamed vegetables. Serves 2

9. CAILY'S SALMON & MISO DISH

Ingredients
- 2 tablespoons miso paste

- 2 tablespoons tamari (wheat-free soy sauce)
- 2 tablespoons apple cider vinegar
- 2 teaspoons grated ginger
- 1/2 teaspoon ground allspice or nutmeg
- Olive oil for greasing pan
- 4 palm-size portions of salmon filets, cut in half
- 1 tablespoon chopped fresh chives

Method
1. Preheat oven to 180°C
2. In a small bowl, whisk miso paste with tamari, apple cider vinegar, ginger, allspice, and one tablespoon of water.
3. Place salmon fillets in a shallow baking pan rubbed lightly with oil.
4. Spoon the miso mixture evenly over the salmon.
5. Broil or grill for 8 to 10 minutes, basting twice or more with marinade, until fish flakes with a fork. Do not overcook.
6. Remove to serving platter. Sprinkle with chopped chives.
7. Serve with three handfuls per serving of steamed greens (beans, broccoli, snow peas, bok choy etc.) drizzled with sesame oil and tamari. Serves 4

10. CLINT'S FISH & PESTO DISH

Ingredients
- 2 palm-size portions of salmon fillets
- 2 tablespoons pesto
- 1 small lemon
- 1 handful of cherry tomatoes
- 1 handful of snow peas, lightly steamed
- 4 handfuls of salad greens, e.g. lettuce, watercress, rocket
- 1 to 2 tablespoons extra virgin olive oil

Method

1. Spread the pesto on both sides of the salmon and cover, and leave to marinate in the fridge for half an hour.
2. After marinating the fish, heat the pan and fry the fish in extra virgin olive oil.
3. Cook fish on both sides until lightly cooked through in the thickest section.
4. Mix salad greens with cherry tomatoes and snow peas and serve with fish.
5. Squeeze lemon juice over fish and salad. Serves 2

11. SALMON & STUFFED CAPSICUMS WITH SALAD

Ingredients
- 2 medium red capsicums
- 80 g feta cheese, crumbled
- 2 eggs
- 1 tablespoon parsley, chopped
- 1 tablespoon basil, chopped
- 1/2 palm size portion of salmon, tinned in brine or spring water

Method
1. Cut capsicums in half lengthways and remove all the seeds and white flesh.
2. In a bowl, mix eggs, feta, herbs and salmon.
3. Fill capsicum halves with this mixture.
4. Bake in the oven for approximately 30 minutes or until set.
5. Serve with two handfuls of allowed vegetables or salad per serve. Serves

12. Fish and Vegetable Stew

Ingredients
- 250 g firm fish fillet
- 2 tbsp lemon juice
- 150 g zucchini
- 250 g eggplant

- 200 g ripe tomatoes
- 1 medium onion
- 1 clove garlic (fine chopped)
- 1 tbsp Olive oil
- 2 tbsp tomato paste
- 300 ml vegetable stock
- Sea Salt to taste
- Pinch of cayenne
- 3 tbsp Soy milk or soft tofu
- tbsp fresh chopped dill (1 tsp dried)

Method
1. Cube the fish and drizzle with half of the lemon juice.
2. Cube all of the vegetables.
3. Marinade the eggplant in the rest of the lemon juice for 10 minutes. Then squeeze them out.
4. Chop up the onion and garlic and saute with the vegetables (except the tomatoes) for 5 minutes.
5. Stir in the tomato paste, then the vegetable stock and bring to a boil.
6. Salt the fish and add to the vegetables and stock, and simmer for 7 minutes.
7. Add the tomatoes and simmer for a further 2 minutes.
8. Stir in the soy milk or the tofu, add a little more lemon juice and adjust the seasoning. Serve with brown rice or rice noodles.

13. Tuna Pie

Ingredients
- 1 tin (450g) tuna or salmon in water 3 eggs
- 1 cup soy milk 1 cup grated tofu
- 1½ cups rice flakes 1 diced onion
- lemon juice

- Mix tuna, lemon juice, onion, tofu and rice flakes.
- Beat eggs and add soy milk then combine with other ingredients.
- Bake in a moderate oven for 45 minutes.

Pie Crust:
- ¾ cup brown rice flour
- ¾ cup millet flakes 5-6 tbsp water
- Mix all ingredients together and press lightly into a grease pie plate or other oven-proof dish.

14. Salmon Patties

Ingredients
- 1 tin (450g) pink salmon
- 2 eggs, lightly beaten
- 1 cup mashed potato
- ½ tsp kelp or parsley
- sprinkle of cayenne pepper
- 1 tbsp lemon juice
- 1 small diced onion
- ¼ cup cold pressed olive oil
- sesame seeds

Method
1. Fork the salmon until flaked.
2. Stir in beaten eggs, potato, seasonings, onion and lemon juice and mix well.
3. Make into patties, pat with sesame seeds and cook in a little oil in a pan until brown on both sides.
4. Alternatively you can cook the patties in the oven until heated through (about 180ºC.)

Chicken

1. ASIAN CHICKEN SOUP

Ingredients
- 2 garlic cloves, finely chopped
- 1 long red chilli, deseeded and finely chopped
- 1 lemongrass stem, white part only, deseeded and finely chopped
- 2 cm cube of fresh ginger, peeled and finely chopped
- 1 handful spring onions, chopped
- 2 tablespoons olive oil
- 1/2 teaspoon sesame oil
- 1-litre chicken stock
- 1 1/2 tablespoons fish sauce
- 2 tablespoon lime juice
- 1 teaspoon Xylitol or Stevia (optional)
- Salt to taste
- 4 palm-size portions of chicken breast, finely sliced
- 4 handfuls mushrooms, sliced
- 4 handfuls bok choy, sliced stems and leaves
- 4 handfuls red capsicum, sliced
- Small handful of coriander leaves, chopped
- 8 basil leaves, chopped

Method
1. Heat olive oil and sesame oil in a heavy-bottomed soup pot. Add garlic, chilli, lemongrass, ginger and spring onions and fry until fragrant (almost browning).
2. Add chicken stock and bring to a boil. Reduce heat to a simmer, and add fish sauce, lime juice, sweetener and salt to taste.
3. Add the chicken and mushrooms and simmer until almost cooked (approximately 5 minutes).
4. Add bok choy stems and capsicum and simmer until tender (approximately 2 minutes). Remove from heat, add bok choy leaves, coriander and basil, stir well and serve in large soup bowls. Serves 4

2. CHICKEN TAJINE WITH PRESERVED LEMON AND OLIVES

Ingredients
Chermoula Marinade
- 2 cloves garlic, chopped
- 1/2 preserved lemon, rinsed and thinly sliced
- 2 onions, chopped
- 1/2 birds eye chilli
- 1 tablespoon sweet paprika
- 1 tablespoon ground cumin
- A pinch of salt
- 2 tablespoons fresh coriander, stems and leaves, chopped
- 2 tablespoons fresh parsley, chopped
- 1/2 teaspoon saffron threads soaked in a bit of water
- 1/2 cup olive oil
- 2 bay leaves, torn in half

Chicken
- 1 whole chicken, size 10 or 12
- 1 tomato, chopped
- 1 onion, chopped
- 2 large leeks, cut into wedges
- 1 onion, sliced
- 1 tomato, sliced
- 150 g pitted green olives
- 1 bunch fresh coriander, chopped
- 1 cup water
- 1 preserved lemon, cut into six segments.

Method
Marinade
1. Process all marinade ingredients together in a food processor until finely chopped and thoroughly combined. Leave for 30 minutes before using. It can be stored in the refrigerator for up to seven days.

2. Wash and dry the chicken and remove the backbone, wing tips, and excess fat. Cut into pieces. Rub all over with 1/2 of the chermoula marinade and refrigerate for at least 2 hours.

Cooking

Combine the tomato and onion with a little of the chermoula marinade and
- Spread into the base of the tajine (this will prevent the chicken from burning on the bottom). Arrange chicken pieces in the centre of the tajine on top of the tomato marinade.
- Coat leek wedges with chermoula and arrange them around the chicken. Top with onion slices, then tomato slices and olives in between the leek wedges.
- Mix chopped coriander with the remaining chermoula marinade and water. Pour over mixture. Decorate the top with preserved lemon wedges.
- Cover tajine with a lid and cook on low heat for 45 minutes. Do not stir or lift the lid during the cooking process.
- Serve one palm-size portion of chicken for each person once cooked. Serve with three handfuls of allowed vegetables or salad per serve.

3. **HOMEMADE CHICKEN SOUP**

Ingredients
- 2 palm-size portions of chicken breast, cubed
- 3 cups chicken stock
- 2 handfuls celery stalks, sliced
- 1 handful onion, chopped
- 1 handful of green beans, chopped
- 1 handful carrot, chopped
- 1 clove garlic
- 1 chilli (optional)
- Chopped parsley to garnish
- 1 tablespoon extra virgin olive oil

Method
1. Lightly fry the onion in olive oil. Add chicken, green beans, carrot, celery, garlic and chilli, sautéing for another minute. Add stock and simmer for 15 minutes. Serves 2

4. CHICKEN WITH A HINT OF PORTUGUESE FLAVOUR

Ingredients
- 1/2 onion, chopped
- 2 small red chillies, deseeded and chopped
- 4 garlic cloves, chopped
- 2 ground bay leaves
- 1/4 teaspoon paprika
- Pinch salt
- 2 teaspoon olive oil (for marinade)
- Juice of 1/2 lemon
- 2 palm-size portions of chicken breast, chopped into large pieces
- 2 teaspoon olive oil (for frying)

Method
1. Blend or crush all ingredients excluding chicken, in a mortar, pestle, or food processor.
2. Marinate chicken in this mixture for at least 30 minutes or overnight if desired.
3. Fry chicken in olive oil until browned and cooked through.
4. Serve with three handfuls of allowed vegetables or salad per serve. Serves 2

5. INDIAN-STYLE CHICKEN WITH SHREDDED CABBAGE

Ingredients
- 2 palm-size portions of chicken breast, diced
- 2 handfuls cabbage, finely shredded
- 2 shallots, finely sliced
- 1 clove garlic, crushed

- 1/4 teaspoon minced ginger
- 1/4 teaspoon ground cumin
- 1/4 teaspoon garam masala
- 1/4 teaspoon fennel seeds
- 1/4 chilli, chopped very finely
- Sea salt and pepper to taste
- 1 tablespoon olive oil

Method
1. Coat chicken with olive oil. Sprinkle with sea salt and pepper to taste. Place under a preheated grill and cook on both sides.
2. Heat pan, add the spices and olive oil, and cook a few seconds before adding shallots. Sauté for a few minutes, then add the shredded cabbage.
3. Cook on high heat for a minute whilst stirring quickly, then reduce the heat to low. Continue to cook until the cabbage has wilted and has been thoroughly coated with spice mixture (you may need to add a little water to moisten). Serve with chicken.
4. Serve with two additional handfuls of allowed vegetables or salad per serve. Serves 2

6. TANDOORI CHICKEN
A traditional Indian-style dish

Ingredients
- 4 palm size portions of chicken breast
- 200 g natural yoghurt (no added sugar)
- 1/2 tablespoon fresh ginger, grated finely
- 1/2 tablespoon garlic, grated finely
- 1/2 tablespoon tandoori paste
- 1 teaspoon cumin seeds, ground
- 1 teaspoon ground coriander
- 1/2 teaspoon garam masala
- 1/4 teaspoon chilli powder
- 1/4 teaspoon turmeric powder
- Salt to taste

Method
1. In a bowl mix together yoghurt, salt, chilli, coriander, cumin, garam masala and tandoori paste. Next, rub the mixture into chicken and leave to marinate for at least 2 hours in the fridge.
2. Preheat the oven to 180°C. Bake chicken for 20 minutes, then reduce the oven heat to 120°C and cook until tender.
3. Garnish with tomatoes and lettuce.
4. Serve with three handfuls of allowed vegetables or salad per serve. Serves 4

7. TROY'S BLACK PEPPER & LEMON CHICKEN

Ingredients
- 3 palm size portions of chicken breast
- 11/4 teaspoons sea salt
- Ground black pepper
- 1/4 cup lemon juice
- 3 teaspoons butter
- 4 teaspoons fresh rosemary, chopped (or 2 teaspoons dried rosemary)
- 2 tablespoons green olives, sliced in half

Method
1. Place chicken between waxed paper or plastic wrap pieces and pound with a large flat knife or meat mallet evenly to 2 cm thick. Sprinkle with salt and pepper.
2. Heat a large frying pan over medium-high heat until hot.
3. Melt butter and sear chicken quickly until browned.
4. Sprinkle with rosemary and add lemon juice and olives. Cook for 2 to 3 minutes or until chicken is well cooked.
5. Serve with three handfuls of allowed vegetables or salad per serve. Serves 3

8. CHICKEN AND TARRAGON PATTIES

Ingredients
- 4 palm size portions of chicken mince
- 1/2 handful red onion, chopped
- 1 tablespoon fresh or dried tarragon leaves, chopped
- 2 teaspoons Dijon mustard
- 1/2 teaspoon sea salt
- Black pepper to taste
- 2 eggs

Method
1. Preheat oven to 180°C. Combine chicken mince with onion, tarragon, mustard, salt, pepper, and eggs in a mixing bowl. Mix thoroughly.
2. Shape into patties. Place on a greased tray.
3. Cook for approximately 10 minutes on each side until browned and cooked through.
4. Serve with three handfuls of allowed vegetables or salad per serve. Serves 4

9. PETA'S CHICKEN DRUMSTICKS

Ingredients
- 6 chicken drumsticks
- 3 tablespoons of soy sauce
- 1 tablespoon crushed garlic
- Olive oil for cooking

Method
1. Cook drumsticks with garlic and soy in a covered pan on low heat until cooked through. Turn regularly. It can be served cold.
2. Serve three drumsticks with three handfuls of allowed vegetables or salad per serve.
   (Drumsticks can be served alone as a snack) Serves 2

10. JULIA'S LEMON CHICKEN

Ingredients
- 1/2 cup lemon juice

- 1 tablespoon soy sauce
- 1 tablespoon mustard
- 1 teaspoon olive oil
- A pinch of cayenne pepper
- 1 palm size portion of chicken breast, diced

Method
1. Combine lemon juice, soy sauce, mustard, olive oil and cayenne pepper. Add the diced chicken and toss around in a bowl to coat well. Leave to marinate for an hour or so if you wish.
2. Heat the pan and fry the chicken. Halfway through frying, turn the chicken over and marinate with more sauce. Cook this side for a further 10 minutes or until cooked.

Serve with three handfuls of allowed vegetables or salad. Serves 1

11. ROASTED CHICKEN

Ingredients
- 2 palm-size portions of chicken breast
- 1/2 cup fresh lemon juice
- Pinch salt
- Pinch black pepper
- Fresh rosemary

Method
1. Preheat oven to 180°C.
2. Marinate chicken breast with lemon juice, rosemary, salt and black pepper for 30 minutes.
3. Place chicken in a shallow baking tray and bake in the oven at 180°C for 10 to 15 minutes or until cooked.
4. Remove the chicken from the baking tray and slice. Set aside.

Serve with three handfuls of allowed vegetables or salad per serve. Serves 2

12. CHICKEN SALSA WITH MEXICAN-STYLE FLAVOUR

Ingredients
- 2 palm-size portions of chicken breast, cut into thin bite-size pieces
- 4 handfuls of mixed broccoli florets and finely sliced green capsicum
- 2 handfuls mushrooms, finely sliced
- 1 clove garlic
- 2 teaspoons tomato paste (no added sugar)
- 1/2 cup water
- 1 teaspoon dried onion flakes
- Tabasco sauce to taste
- Sea salt and cracked pepper to taste
- Olive oil for cooking
- A sprinkling of Italian seasoning
- Garnishing of fresh chopped parsley

Method
1. To make salsa, mix water, tomato paste, tabasco sauce, sea salt, pepper and onion flakes and let stand.
2. Coat the frying pan with olive oil. Over moderate heat, add crushed garlic, chicken, mushrooms, broccoli and green capsicum. Mix and toss until chicken is browned, then add tomato salsa mixture, stirring well until evenly mixed through.
3. When ready to serve, sprinkle over with parsley.

13. GREEN CURRY CHICKEN & VEGETABLES

Ingredients
- 2 palm-size portions of chicken breast
- 1 tablespoon extra virgin olive oil
- Green curry paste (no added sugar)
- 1 medium onion
- Finely chopped ginger to taste
- 1/2 cup of coconut milk (low-fat)

- 3 handfuls each of lightly steamed broccoli, beans, and zucchini, cut lengthways

Method
1. Cut the chicken breast into strips, slice the onion into rings and sauté with ginger in olive oil until the chicken is cooked.
2. Add coconut milk and green curry paste. Simmer for 5 to 10 minutes.
3. Serve alongside steamed vegetables. Serves 2

14. WOK STYLED GINGER CHICKEN

Ingredients
- 2 palm-size portions of chicken breast, cut into small cubes
- 1/2 handful onion, cut lengthwise
- 2 handfuls red capsicum, cut into strips
- 2 handfuls celery stalks, cut diagonally
- 2 teaspoons grated ginger
- 1/2 handful of blanched almonds
- 1 handful of bamboo shoots
- 1 handful of snow peas
- Extra virgin olive oil for cooking

Method
1. Add extra virgin olive oil to a wok and cook almonds until golden. Remove and drain on absorbent paper.
2. Add 1 teaspoon ginger, sauté for 1 minute, then add all vegetables. Cook for 1 to 2 minutes and place to side.
3. Place chicken and remaining ginger in a pan, with a little more oil and cook until almost done. Return vegetables and almonds to the pan and warm through. Serves 2

15. TURKEY FILLET WITH RED CABBAGE

Ingredients
- 2 palm-size portions of Turkey fillet

- 3 handfuls red cabbage, finely sliced
- 1 handful onion
- 2 handfuls apple, finely sliced
- 3 cloves
- 1 teaspoon cider vinegar
- Olive oil for cooking

Method
1. Bake the barbeque turkey fillet for approximately 25-30 minutes.
2. In a pan with a lid, sauté onion in a bit of olive oil for 1 minute. Add cabbage and cook for another minute. Add apple slices and cloves.
3. Seal the pan tightly and reduce heat. Simmer for 20 minutes. Two minutes before the end of cooking, add vinegar.
4. Serve cabbage on a plate; place cooked turkey fillet on cabbage. Serves 2

Lamb

1. AUSSIE-STYLE WINTER STEW

Ingredients
- 2 palm-size portions of lamb or beef, diced or cubed
- 1 tablespoon of butter
- Pinch salt
- 2 teaspoons parsley
- 2 teaspoons Worcestershire sauce
- 1/2 handful onion, chopped
- 2 cloves garlic
- 1 handful of broccoli, diced
- 2 handfuls turnips, diced
- 1 handful carrot, diced
- 1 handful of cauliflower, diced
- 1/2 handful of mushroom, diced
- 250 ml beef or vegetable stock

Method
Brown meat in melted butter. Add seasonings and Worcestershire sauce. Place all ingredients into a casserole dish and cook in a moderate oven until meat and vegetables are tender. Serves 2

2. LAMB AND EGGPLANT CURRY

Ingredients
- 2 handfuls eggplant, cut in half lengthways, sliced
- 2 tablespoons olive oil
- 1 large onion, thinly sliced
- 2 palm-size portions of lamb fillet, diced
- 3 teaspoons green curry paste (no added sugar)
- 2 kaffir lime leaves
- 200 mL coconut milk (low fat)
- 2 handfuls of baby green beans
- 2 tablespoons soy sauce
- 2 tablespoons fish sauce
- 2 handfuls baby spinach leaves

Method
1. Sprinkle eggplant with salt and set aside for 30 minutes. Rinse, squeeze and dry in a tea towel.
2. Heat oil in a wok. When hot, add eggplant and fry over high heat for 1 to 2 minutes until golden. Drain on a paper towel. Add onion to wok and fry for 1 to 2 minutes.
3. Add lamb and cook for 1 minute, then add the curry paste and lime leaves. Cook over high heat for a few seconds.
4. Return eggplant to wok with coconut milk and beans. Bring to the boil. Add soy sauce, fish sauce and spinach, stirring to wilt spinach. Serve hot. Serves 2

3. BBQ LAMB SKEWERS

Ingredients
- 2 tablespoons sour cream (low fat)
- 2 tablespoons lemon juice

- 2 tablespoons capers, drained, chopped
- 1 garlic clove, crushed
- 4 palm size portions of lamb backstrap, cubed
- 2 handfuls mushrooms, halved
- 2 handfuls capsicums, cut into small pieces
- Olive oil cooking spray
- 2 tablespoons fresh rosemary, chopped

Method
1. Combine sour cream, lemon juice, capers and garlic in a bowl. Set aside.
2. Thread the lamb, mushrooms and capsicum onto eight pre-soaked skewers. Spray with olive oil. Sprinkle with rosemary.
3. Preheat a barbecue plate or chargrill on medium heat. Cook skewers, turning occasionally, for 6 to 8 minutes or until browned and cooked to your liking. Remove to a plate. Set aside, covered, for 5 minutes to rest.
4. Serve with two additional handfuls of allowed vegetables or salad per serve. Serves 4

4. VEGETABLES & LAMB CUTLETS

Ingredients
- 2 palm-size portions of lean lamb cutlets
- 2 handfuls each of cauliflower, broccoli florets and green beans
- 1 teaspoon Worcestershire sauce
- 1/2 teaspoon vinegar
- 1/4 teaspoon onion powder
- 1/4 teaspoon French mustard
- 2 tablespoons water
- Sea salt and freshly ground pepper
- Fresh chopped parsley and chives
- 1 teaspoon slivered almonds

Method

1. Steam cauliflower, broccoli florets and green beans on low heat until tender. Set aside.
2. Mix Worcestershire sauce, vinegar, onion, mustard, sea salt and pepper with water.
3. Baste each side of the cutlet with the sauce mixture. Then coat each side lightly with olive oil. Place under a preheated grill and grill each side until cooked.
4. Serve with steamed vegetables and garnish with freshly chopped parsley, chives and slivered almonds. Serves 2

5. MARINATED LAMB BACKSTRAP

Ingredients
- 4 palm-size portions of lamb back strap, cut into 2 cm strips

Marinade
- 1/2 tablespoon cumin
- 1/2 tablespoon sweet paprika
- Salt
- 1 tablespoon chopped garlic
- 1/2 tablespoon coriander leaves, chopped
- 1/2 tablespoon continental parsley, chopped
- 1/2 tablespoon lemon juice
- A good drizzle of olive oil

Method
1. Put lamb into a bowl and add all the marinade ingredients. Use your hands to combine. Cover and leave for 1 hour in the fridge before grilling medium/rare on the barbecue.
2. Serve with three handfuls of allowed vegetables or salad per serve. Serves 4

Turkey

1. Thai Style Turkey Salad

*For the **turkey** component:*
Allow a maximum of 100 g of turkey per person.

Gently grill (preferable) or pan-fry the turkey schnitzels or steaks and season with sea salt. When done, cut into strips and reserve.

*For the **salad** take:*
- 2 cups Baby spinach
- 2 cups Asian Greens
- 2 cup fine cut Chinese cabbage
- 1 cup Snow or Sugar snap peas, cut into strips 1 small Lebanese cucumber
- Handful of coriander minced Handful of Mint, minced
- 2 tbsp Toasted sesame seeds
- Handful of spring onion tops, minced
- For the dressing:
- 2 tbsp hulled Tahini (sesame paste)
- 1 tbsp of sunflower or canola oil
- 2 tsp minced garlic 1 tsp minced ginger 1 lemon as juice
- 1 tsp fine grated lemon rind (yellow part only)
- 2 tbsp water
- 2 tbsp of Braggs or light soy sauce 2 tsp honey (softened)
- 1 pinch cayenne 1/5 tsp sea salt

Method
1. Place the ingredients in a jar and shake or process until blended.
2. Mix the salad greens with the herbs, the peas and as much of the dressing as needed. Sprinkle with toasted sesame seeds, and serve with the turkey strips scattered over the top.

Beef

1. GRILLED PEPPER STEAK WITH BEANS AND SAUCE

Ingredients
- 2 palm-size portions of sirloin or fillet steak
- 2 tablespoons extra virgin olive oil
- Freshly ground black pepper
- 6 handfuls French or green beans

<u>Lemon butter sauce</u>
- 60 grams organic butter
- Juice of 1/2 a freshly squeezed lemon
- Freshly ground black pepper

Method
1. Brush steaks with olive oil on both sides and season liberally with black pepper—place under a hot grill, at least 8 cm from heat, and grill to taste.
2. While the steak is grilling, steam the beans until tender but still firm. Heat the butter in a small saucepan, stir in the lemon juice and freshly ground pepper.
3. Serve steaks with beans, pouring the sauce over beans. Serves 2

2. GRILLED STEAK WITH A SIDE OF GARLIC ZUCCHINI
Keep it simple

Ingredients
- 1 palm-size portion of steak
- 2 handfuls zucchini, sliced
- 4 tablespoons of water
- 1 small clove garlic, crushed
- Fresh chopped parsley
- Olive oil cooking spray
- Sea salt
- Cracked pepper

Method
1. Drizzle olive oil over the steak. Sprinkle with sea salt and cracked pepper. Grill under a preheated grill and cook as desired.
2. Spray coat a small saucepan with olive oil cooking spray. Sauté garlic and add water. Gently toss zucchini slices and cook until tender. Garnish with fresh parsley.

Serve with one additional handful of allowed vegetables or salad. Serves 1

3. THAI-STYLE STIR-FRY

Ingredients
- 2 palm-size portions of beef, diced
- 1 1/2 tablespoons sesame oil
- 1 1/2 handfuls bean sprouts
- 1 clove garlic
- 1 teaspoon minced ginger
- 1 1/2 handfuls snow peas
- 1 1/2 handfuls red capsicum, sliced
- 1 1/2 handfuls mushrooms, sliced
- 1/2 cup flaked almonds
- 1 1/2 tablespoons lemon/lime juice
- 1 1/2 tablespoons soy sauce

Method
1. Sauté beef with ginger, garlic and soy sauce until brown.
2. Add vegetables and cook for 2 to 3 minutes.
3. Sprinkle almonds over a meal just before serving.
4. Dress with lime juice and sesame oil. Serves 2

4. MOROCCAN MEAT PATTIES

Ingredients
- 1 handful onion, chopped
- 1 large green chilli, finely chopped
- 3 to 4 cloves garlic, finely chopped

- 1 teaspoon ground sweet paprika
- 1/2 teaspoon ground turmeric
- 1/2 teaspoon ground cumin
- 1 handful tomato, blanched in hot water, peeled and chopped
- 4 handfuls zucchini, grated
- 1/2 preserved lemon (rind only), or zest of 1/2 lemon, chopped (if using lemon zest, add an additional pinch of salt)
- 4 palm size portions of lean beef mince
- 2 eggs, lightly beaten
- Few sprigs each of fresh mint, coriander leaves and parsley
- Salt and pepper to taste
- Olive oil

Method
- Fry the onion with olive oil for a few minutes until almost transparent. Add green chilli, garlic, paprika, turmeric and cumin, and fry for a further few minutes. Add tomato, preserved lemon (or zest) zucchini and cook for 4 to 5 minutes or until zucchini is tender and some liquid evaporates.
- In a large bowl, combine the cooked mixture with beef mince, eggs, herbs, salt and pepper. Mix well and shape into small patties. Fry the meat patties in olive oil, turning gently, until cooked through and lightly browned on both sides.
- Serve with two additional handfuls of allowed vegetables or salad per serve. Serves 4

5. SPICY MEATBALLS & VEGGIES

Ingredients
Meatballs
- 4 palm size portions of lean beef mince
- 1 onion, chopped finely
- 2 cloves garlic, chopped finely
- 1/2 teaspoon cumin
- 1/2 teaspoon paprika

- 2 teaspoons olive oil
- 1/2 handful parsley, chopped
- 2 eggs
- 1/2 teaspoon lemon zest
- Salt and pepper to taste

Stock
- 1 cup chicken stock
- 1/2 teaspoon lemon zest
- 1/2 teaspoon cumin
- 1/2 teaspoon turmeric

Vegetables
3 handfuls per serving of seasonal green vegetables, e.g. green beans, zucchini, broccoli, and snow peas. (12 handfuls in total)

Method
1. Fry onion, garlic and spices in 1 teaspoon olive oil. Add to mince with lemon zest, eggs, herbs, salt and pepper.
2. Mix well and shape into small, golf ball size balls. Heat 1 teaspoon olive oil and cook the meatballs for 1 to 2 minutes until sealed.
3. Heat stock with spices and lemon zest. Add stock to meatballs and simmer until cooked through and stock thickens to a sauce. Add more stock if required through the cooking process to keep it moist.
4. Serve with sauce on a bed of freshly steamed green vegetables. Serves 4

AFTER-DINNER SNACKS

OK, we have all fallen into the trap of snacking after dinner. It's my personal danger time, sitting there happily relaxed, (or lonely or bored) watching TV when my mind wanders to the fridge, chocolates or cookie jar. So here are some suggestions to help.

Practical Advice

It is best not to eat after dinner. However, make it healthy if you have to eat something in the evenings. So although it's best not to overeat after meals if you have to, then try the following recommendations:

- **CHICKEN LEG SNACK**

Great to have when craving carbs and want a quick snack

Ingredients
- 6 chicken drumsticks
- 2 tablespoons of lemon grass chopped
- 1 tablespoon crushed garlic
- 3 kaffir lime leaves
- Olive oil for cooking

Method
Cook drumsticks with garlic and kaffir lime, chilli and lemongrass in a covered pan on low heat until cooked. Turn regularly. It can be served cold.
Serves six snacks

- If you have an air fryer, this would be an even quicker way to prepare the six chicken legs and healthier as it saves frying.

My preferred method of cooking the chicken legs.
Salt to taste the legs with Himalayan rock salt and sprinkle with black seed pepper (Nigella Sativa). Lightly coat the legs with garlic paste.
Air fry until cooked, and eat one leg while hot and the rest later cold.

- **VEGGIE CHIPS**

Ingredients
- 3 handfuls eggplant, cut into 3 to 5 mm slices
- 3 handfuls zucchinis, cut diagonally into 3 to 5 mm slices

- 2 handfuls fennel, peeled, halved and cut into 3 to 5 mm slices
- 1 1/2 handfuls green beans, snapped and halved
- 1 tablespoon olive oil
- 2 teaspoons tamari (wheat-free soy sauce)

Method
1. Cut eggplant first. As some larger eggplants may be bitter, toss slices with one teaspoon salt and then let them sit while preparing other vegetables to draw out the bitter liquid. Rinse off briny liquid and pat slices dry.
2. Place equal-sized, dry vegetable slices in a large mixing bowl. Pour oil and tamari over vegetable slices, tossing to coat evenly.
3. Place coated slices in a food dehydrator or on a lightly greased tray. Dehydrate at 45 degrees for 4 to 8 hours or at the oven's lowest setting for 3 to 4 hours until vegetables are dried and crunchy, leathery or chewy crunchy.
4. Cool and serve as a snack or with soup.

You can use any vegetables, e.g. cauliflower, celery, and green beans.
Serves 3 (Vegetable Side Dish)

Other food choices you can add occasionally
- Shirataki Noodle
- Kelp Noodles - A sea vegetable? It looks like a noodle & Tastes like one too!

Chapter Seven

This Diet Plan Makes Socialising Easy and Enjoyable.

- ❖ The wonderful thing about this diet plan is that you can eat a wide variety of foods, and most café and restaurants will have allowed foods. Even some fast food places serve grilled chicken and salads. Just say NO to the fries and soft drink. You can order fish or chicken and even a steak. But order a small or even an entree-size meal.
- ❖ Order your meal without dangerous foods (e.g. chips, potato, rice etc.). It is easier to avoid it if it is not on your plate.
- ❖ Ask for all dressings/sauces to be served on the side. Substitute creamy salad dressings for vinaigrette. Be aware of the hidden ingredients and sugars that can be included in many sauces.
- ❖ Assess serving sizes in relation to your palm size and approximate handfuls. Rule of thumb a piece of meat should be about the size of the palm of your hand. If the servings are too large, ask for a side plate to place excess food on and have it taken away immediately.
- ❖ Drink Green Tea or black coffee and still be able to meet friends at cafés.
- ❖ If you cannot resist ordering something for dessert, try ordering a black coffee or go for the cheese platter instead of cake/sweets.
- ❖ Avoid buffet and 'all you can eat' style restaurants.
- ❖ Avoid alcohol.
- ❖ Ask for a bottle or jug of water for the table and drink that instead of soft drinks, juices or alcohol.

Bon appetite...

Summary:

You don't stay on this Diet forever – it's designed for 6-8 weeks at a time. It also helps to change and enjoy other foods not on this diet plan at rotational times.

Philip's Guide to continued health and healing
I suggest you read my book series to gain knowledge and wisdom for a long-term lifestyle of health, happiness and enjoying food. You are free to eat whatever you want, your body is your responsibility, and I know that now you have read this book, you will choose well. I am also available for consultations both locally and long distance.

What to do next?
First, compare the records of how you were before and after the program. Congratulate yourself on the changes, no matter how large or small they may be. Appreciate the changes you have been able to create in such a short time.
The next step is to keep the momentum going to reach your goals, and I offer the following to help you achieve just that.

1. Daniels Diet

If you need more help in weight loss or want to freshen your body to feel clean and energised. Then this is the ideal diet plan for this. Lots of fruit and Veggies on this Diet – very effective and healthy for you.

2. Daniels Diet Recipe Guide.

This recipe book is a vegetarian (vegan) food plan. Two incredible Christian chefs and I specifically created it.

3. Quick & Fast Meals – A 7-Day Eating Plan for 'The Busy Women'. With easy and fast recipes – all under 15 minutes.

About the Author

Philip's interest in studying natural therapies has spanned most of his adult life. As a practitioner with expertise in various professional fields, he has more than 30 years of successful clinical practice, a wealth of knowledge and extensive firsthand experience of the profound benefits of natural therapies.

Highly qualified, Philip's formal qualifications include a Bachelor of Science (BSc) in Health, a Diploma in Naturopathy (ND), a post-graduate Diploma in Herbal Medicine, and an Associate Diploma in Theology.

With his theory of 'Food for Medicine,' he helped pioneer the establishment and expansion of modern-day Natural Therapies within Western Australia.

In 1985, Philip wrote a Book on Chronic Fatigue Syndrome. This was one of the first books ever written on Chronic Fatigue by a practitioner. For his research in this area, he was nominated for the 'Australian Pursuit of Excellence Award.'
And he had two books published internationally:
1. Daniels Diet –best seller and American Award Winning book
2. Daniels Diet Lifestyle,

In the recent past, Philip was the Feature writer for health columns in three magazines and, for five years, was the weekly guest Naturopath on a radio segment in Perth.

A highly proficient presenter, Philip encompasses both practical and spiritual subject matters and is available to speak at business meetings, professional associations and church groups. He regularly travels across Australia and Singapore communicating the message of Health and wholeness.

Philip's private naturopathic practice is located in Western Australia. Private consultations are available, both in person and for overseas and interstate people, through long-distance consultation via Zoom, Skype or Phone.

For further information, visit:
www.wisdomforhealth.com

Philip would like to thank Metagenics Australia for freely sharing their recipes and ideas in this Diet Plan.

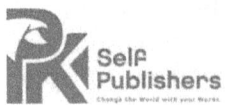

PK – SELF PUBLISHING

How do I get my book written and published?

We can do it all for you!! I wish someone had made me this offer 20 years ago when I wrote my first book, it just makes things so much easier, and you get it done 'now', not years later.

You know you have a story to tell and a message to share. You want to tell your story and impact the world, but you're unsure how to get it published. There are many steps to take to get from start to finish, and many people are just too busy to be able to do the necessary time-consuming work involved.

The good news is that we can help you turn your story, testimony, biography, sermons, teaching, expertise or business ideas into your finished book.

1. We offer to take your book from sitting in a file on your computer to a professionally finished book.
2. We will process your Word doc or PDF file into the most popular professional formats such as EBooks and printed Paperback Books
EBooks: compatible with all major book retailers, including Amazon, Barnes and noble, Apple iBooks and much more.
3. Arguably, one of the more frustrating areas of creating a Book (post-composition) is making sure that your book is formatted, converted and distributed worldwide.
4. We can also professionally edit, proofread and critique if needed.
5. We do your book covers designing and more...

Testimony from our last two clients

CW: *Without Philip and Kriste's help, I would not have finished my book, let alone get it published on Amazon. Now I am selling it literally all over the world. I have been invited to talk on the radio and to give a talk at my university. Doors are opening to me that I would never have before my book. Don't wait – get them to help you – it's worth it, and they are great to work with too.*

Leigh: *Hi Philip and Kriste, I am so excited, I went onto Amazon, and it said #1 Bestseller besides our book when I looked at it this morning! Thank you so much for helping me write and publish my book. I remember I only had my rough manuscript draft when I first spoke to you. You took it from there to a professional-level book, and now I Am an Author...WOW, it would have taken me years to do it myself.*

If you have questions and you know you have a book to write but need help to get it done, contact us, and we will encourage and give our initial guidance for FREE... Email us at **thebridgemanway@gmail.com**

DANIEL'S DIET AND
Working With Jesus For Your Health

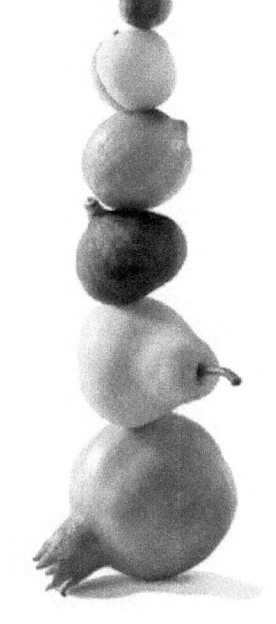

THE 10 DAY WEIGHT LOSS AND DETOX PLAN

A biblical diet program that's been successful for over 2000 years and will work for you.

PHILIP BRIDGEMAN BSc, ND.

www.ingramcontent.com/pod-product-compliance
Lightning Source LLC
Chambersburg PA
CBHW060032040426
42333CB00042B/2371